an introduction to

reiki

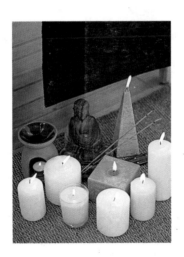

an introduction to
reiki

healing energy for
mind, body and spirit

mary lambert

consultant: chris parkes, usui master

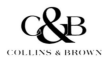

COLLINS & BROWN

safety note

*Reiki should never be considered as a substitute for medical treatment.
It can be practised in conjunction with it, with a few exceptions (see
page 33), but a doctor should always be consulted in regard to worrying
symptoms that require diagnosis. The author and publishers cannot be held
liable for any errors or omissions in this book or for any actions that may be
taken as a consequence of using it.*

First published in Great Britain in 2000
by Collins & Brown Limited
London House
Great Eastern Wharf
Parkgate Road
London SW11 4NQ

Distributed in the United States and Canada by Sterling Publishing Co,
387 Park Avenue South, New York, NY 10016, USA

Copyright © Collins & Brown Limited 2000

Text copyright © Mary Lambert 2000
Photographs copyright © Collins & Brown 2000, except for pages 9 and 13,
© Phyllis Lei Furumoto, and pages 84–87, 90 © The Photographers' Library

The right of Mary Lambert to be identified as the author of this work has been
asserted by her in accordance with the Copyright, Designs and Patents Act, 1988.

9 8 7 6 5 4 3 2 1

British Library Cataloguing-in-Publication Data:
A catalogue record for this book
is available from the British Library.

ISBN 1 85585 747 2

Designer: Sue Miller
Photography: Winfried Heinze

Reproduction by Classic Scan, Singapore
Printed and bound in Italy by New Interlitho

introduction

Reiki (which is pronounced ray-key) is a Japanese word that means "universal life force energy". It is an ancient hands-on healing art that was re-introduced in the mid-19th century by Dr Mikao Usui in Japan. A holistic healing system, reiki works to create spiritual, mental and physical harmony.

The word reiki is composed of two parts: "rei" which defines the universal side of the energy and "ki" which is the life-force energy that flows through every living thing. This concept is found in most cultures under different names – the Chinese call it "chi", the Indian Hindus "prana" and the Christians "light".

healing energy

Reiki is a safe, non-intrusive healing energy which channels itself to wherever it is needed in your body or the person you are treating. By stimulating the body's natural healing ability at the deepest level, it removes physical and emotional blockages that may have been causing illness or upset for some time. The essence of reiki is to cleanse the body and balance the chakras (see pages 24–25), bringing harmony to mind, body and spirit through a detoxifying process as well as promoting a more positive attitude. Reiki differs from other healing methods because of its attunement procedure and the fact that the energy originates from the "universal source" rather than directly from the healer.

Many different ailments can be cured or relieved by reiki. Problems such as headaches, back ache and stress-related illness all respond well to reiki. Chronic illnesses, such as arthritis or asthma, will also benefit from reiki, but require repeated treatments for an improvement to be seen.

This book is for people to use as a reference aid after they have completed First Degree Reiki (Reiki I). It also serves as an introduction to reiki for those who are interested in reiki and want to learn more about its special healing powers. The system of reiki discussed here is the traditional Usui system, as founded and taught by Dr Usui. Other branches of reiki which have developed from students of Usui are Karuna™, which deals with emotional healing, and Tera-Mai Seichem™ which incorporates variations of the traditional teaching style.

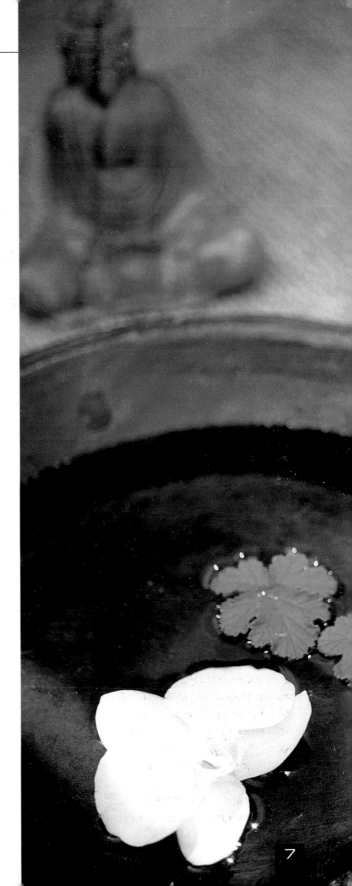

Water plays a large part in the cleansing process of reiki healing.

the three degrees of reiki

Access to this reiki energy is through a series of attunements at First Degree (Reiki I), Second Degree (Reiki II) and Third Degree (Reiki III) initiations (see pages 18–20). This book is mainly concerned with introducing beginners to reiki and those who have taken First Degree Reiki. This is normally done over a weekend, during which the initiates are attuned to the energy by a reiki master so that they can channel it to themselves and also to treat other people. Once a person is attuned, the ability to channel energy stays with them for life.

If you have not been attuned, you can gain some benefit from working through the positions on pages 36–59, just not to the same degree as people who have had the training.

finding a reiki master

The best way to find a reiki master to teach and attune you is through personal recommendation. Alternatively, you can use advertisements in health magazines or shops, but it can be more unpredictable. You can then get in touch with the master concerned and perhaps even have an introductory talk. Small teaching groups are best, but the crucial factor is whether you feel you can bond with the master.

The Second Degree is for people who want to progress further with reiki and intensify the emotional and mental healing they can give by using the reiki symbols and send absent healing (see pages 16–17). The Third Degree initiation is the training and apprenticeship to become a reiki master – this is a spiritual path and lifelong commitment and not something to be undertaken lightly. Reiki healing can, however, be practised at all levels, to treat yourself, friends and family at home or on a more professional level. It will always work to your highest good.

the history of reiki

The story of how this ancient healing was re-discovered by Dr Mikao Usui is told by each reiki master to his students as part of their training at First Degree Reiki (see pages 18–19). This oral tradition has been passed on from master to student for many years, although written versions of the story are now also included in books on reiki. No one questioned the traditional story until some masters, eager to find out more about the origins of reiki, discovered some anomalies in the story being taught, but the essential facts of the story remain the same.

Dr Mikao Usui lived in Kyoto in Japan in the mid-19th century. The country had become more open to foreigners and Dr Usui was converted to Christianity by missionaries, becoming a minister as well as a teacher of the faith. He was the dean of a small Christian university and regularly taught the students. During one of his lessons one of them asked if he believed that the stories in the bible were accurate. He replied that he thought they were. The students continued with their questioning enquiring if he believed in the healing miracles of Christ. When he replied "Yes", the students then wanted to know that as Christ had said "You will do as I have done, and even greater things" why there were not more healers in the world. They then asked if he could teach them the healing methods of Christ. When Dr Usui reluctantly said he could not, his Japanese sense of honour compelled him to resign from his position as dean as he felt he had failed to help his students.

dr usui's quest
Intrigued by his students' last question Dr Usui felt he should try and find out more about Christ's special healing powers. This research in the end became his life's quest. As he had been taught by Western missionaries he decided to begin his research in a Christian country, so he visited the USA. He enrolled at the University of Chicago and studied there for seven years. During this time he received a doctorate in theology, but still did not succeed in finding out how Jesus had managed to heal people.

He decided to return to Japan thinking that he might be able to find out more about the healing methods used by Buddha through studying Buddhism. Travelling around the country he visited several Buddhist monasteries, where he was discouraged in his researches by the monks who said that the focus of Buddhist healing was not on physical healing, but on healing the spirit. However, Dr Usui was determined to continue his search and eventually ended up at a Zen monastery in Kyoto. The abbot of this monastery agreed with him that it must be possible to heal the body as well as the spirit, but the process of physical healing had been lost or forgotten over the years.

Dr Usui spent many years at the monastery studying the Japanese Buddhist scriptures, the sutras, but still could find no useful information. As Buddhism had reached Japan through China, he also learned

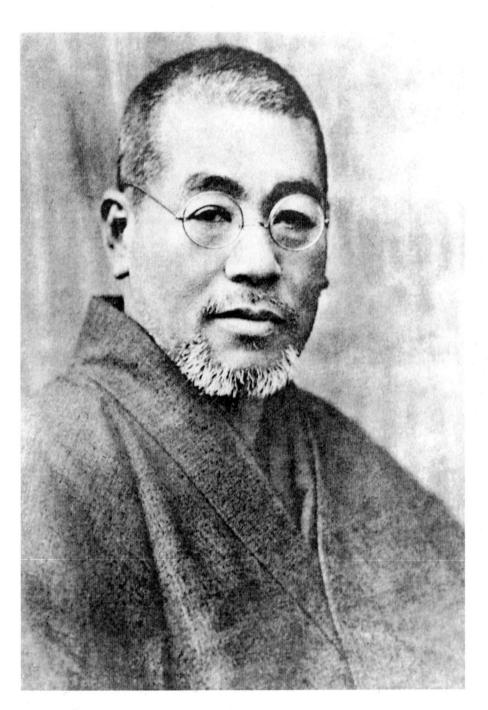

Dr Mikao Usui,
who founded reiki
in the mid-19th
century in Japan.

Chinese to read more sutras. He later went on to study Sanskrit, the ancient Indian language, so that he could also read the Tibetan sutras. After some time he was said to have made a trip to northern India and possibly Tibet. Here he was believed to have read Tibetan scrolls, found in his lifetime, that recounted the journeys of St Isa, who was thought to have been Jesus. Some of the answers he sought were found in the Japanese sutras and some other scripts which described Buddha's healing method, but despite all his travels and research, he could still not make the technique work.

the mountain retreat

Dr Usui returned to the Zen monastery, where he discussed his situation with the abbot. They decided that he should go on a 21-day retreat in the mountains where he would fast and meditate to seek enlightenment. The place chosen for the retreat was a sacred mountain called Mount Kuri Yama, 15–18 miles outside Kyoto. Dr Usui climbed the mountain and chose a special place for his meditation, facing east. He collected 21 stones so that he could keep track of the days by throwing away a stone a day. For 20 days he experienced nothing out of the ordinary, but just before dawn on the 21st day as Dr Usui prayed for a sign, he saw a light appear in the darkness, which grew in size as it approached him. He began to feel very frightened and wanted to run away, but he resisted this impulse as he also felt that he should stay and see if this light would finally give him an answer to his quest.

The light came closer and closer until it struck him in the middle of his forehead. Dr Usui thought he was dying as he saw millions of rainbow-coloured bubbles. The bubbles then slowly changed into white bubbles, and each one contained a Sanskrit character (a reiki symbol) in gold that he had discovered in the Tibetan scripts. Each bubble appeared before him one at a time, so that he could study each character before it disappeared. He was given the meaning of each one and how it could be used to stimulate healing energy. This was the first miracle.

When Dr Usui came round from what had felt like a trance, he found that it was now broad daylight. He started walking down the mountain, anxious to share his experiences with the abbot. As he rushed down, he tripped on a stone and cut his toe. Instinctively, he bent down to hold his toe with his hand and was astonished a few minutes later to find that the bleeding had stopped and the pain had diminished – an amazing healing had taken place. This was the second miracle.

Dr Usui continued to descend and stopped for refreshment at an outdoor inn near the foot of the mountain. He ordered a traditional Japanese breakfast, despite the advice of the proprietor who felt he ought to eat something lighter after such a long fast. When the meal was served he ate it hurriedly, but suffered no discomfort at all. As he was eating, he noticed that the proprietor's granddaughter had a swollen jaw and was suffering from acute toothache. She had not been able to go into town, which was several days' journey away, to see a dentist so Dr Usui asked if he could try and help. When he put his hands over the painful area, the swelling rapidly reduced and the pain disappeared. This was the third miracle of the day.

He continued his journey back to the Zen monastery and on his arrival found the abbot in great pain from arthritis. Once again the doctor put his hands on the affected areas, and to the abbot's amazement, the pain disappeared – the fourth miracle had occurred.

'Reiki will guide you.

Let the reiki hands find it. They will

know what to do.'

(Mrs Hawayo Takata)

helping others

The next day Dr Usui talked to the abbot about how he could best use his new-found healing skill and they decided he should work in the beggars' quarter of Kyoto and help to relieve their suffering. He left the monastery straightaway and went to live with the beggars for several years, healing people and encouraging them to start a new life. However, after some years he realized that many of the beggars, who had been healed and had started afresh, returned to begging. This distressed Dr Usui and he realized that although he had healed the body, he had not healed the spirit as the monks had told him and the beggars were not taking any responsibility for their lives. He began to understand that an exchange of energy was crucial and that people needed to give something back for the healing they had received, so that their lives would not be without value.

Dr Usui left the beggars' quarter and, using the symbols that he had been given (see pages 16–17), taught reiki healing throughout Japan. He also developed the five spiritual principles to complement the physical healing (see pages 14–15) and began to teach people how to treat themselves and others.

the new masters

Dr Usui also started to train other men as masters, and one of these was Dr Chujiro Hayashi, a retired naval officer. The two men worked together for many years, developing the teaching system, and in the early 1920s Dr Usui chose Dr Hayashi as his successor to carry on the tradition of reiki. Dr Hayashi went on to found a reiki clinic in Tokyo where he treated many people, going to their homes if they could not visit the clinic. It was to this clinic that Hawayo Takata, a Japanese-American woman, came to be treated.

Hawayo Takata

Hawayo Takata was born in 1900 on the Hawaiian island of Kauai. In 1935, after being widowed and trying to cope with two small active daughters, she developed depression as well as physical disorders. She was told she needed an operation to save her life, and while visiting her parents in Japan arranged to have the necessary surgery. On the day of the operation as she was being prepared for the operating theatre she heard the voice of her late husband telling her repeatedly that she should not go ahead. Mrs Takata then talked to her doctor about her doubts over this treatment and asked whether there were any other options. The doctor told her about a reiki clinic nearby where a member of his family had been successfully treated.

Mrs Takata went to the clinic for treatment and, although at first sceptical of the sessions, she began to relax and enjoy the healing energy. However, she was amazed by the heat that came out of the hands of her healers and kept looking for electrical equipment that was generating the heat, before they convinced her it was the force of the energy. After several months she was cured. Impressed by the effects of reiki she asked Dr Hayashi if he would teach her the healing method so that she could take it back to Hawaii. Initially she was refused because she was a foreigner and a woman, but eventually Dr Hayashi took her on as an apprentice and during her year's training initiated her in First and Second Degree Reiki (see pages 18–21). Mrs Takata returned to her home in Hawaii and started giving regular reiki sessions. In 1938 she was made a master by Dr Hayashi when he visited her in Hawaii.

Shortly after Dr Hayashi's return to Japan, Mrs Takata had a worrying dream and knew at once that she had to go and see him. When she arrived Dr Hayashi, who also had a similar prophetic experience, talked with her about the likely war between Japan and the United States. He also expressed his concerns that as an ex-naval officer he might be called up for military service. He predicted correctly the outcome of the war and decided to make Mrs Takata his successor as the Grand Master so that he could pass on his knowledge to her and entrust her with continuing the reiki tradition. Shortly after their conversation, just before the start of the war, Dr Hayashi died.

The Usui Grand Master

Mrs Takata returned to Hawaii and continued to practise reiki throughout the war years. During the

40 years after the war she succeeded in bringing reiki to the USA, but it was not until the last ten years of her life when she was in her 70s that she started to train other reiki masters. At the time of her death on 11 December 1980 she had initiated 22 masters to spread reiki throughout the USA and Europe. No successor was named as the Grand Master, but her granddaughter, Phyllis Lei Furomoto, and another Master, Dr Barbara Weber Ray, joined together to promote the Usui system of reiki. However, the two women did not work together for long, and Dr Barbara Weber Ray soon left to found another branch of reiki. A year after Mrs Takata's death many of the elected masters met to form the Reiki Alliance to preserve the reiki tradition and to standardize its teaching practices. They asked Phyllis Lei Furomoto to be the Grand Master of the Usui system, a position she still holds. The Alliance currently has offices in the USA and Europe.

Until early 1988 only the Grand Master could initiate students to be masters. But then Phyllis Lei Furumoto changed the system, allowing all masters to train and initiate people to the Third Degree, so that the knowledge of the traditional Usui system could be spread even further afield.

reiki today

All of the current Usui masters teach the form of reiki passed on by Mrs Takata and Phyllis Lei Furomoto. This contains nine special elements which include initiations, money, symbols, treatments, oral tradition and spiritual lineage. If any of these elements are changed or altered at all, the system is then no longer considered to be Usui.

In the early 1990s, Paul David Mitchell became the head of the Reiki Alliance and works with Phyllis Lei Furomoto to train and advise to masters on interpreting the Usui elements throughout the world, ensuring that all the Usui reiki training conforms to their standards.

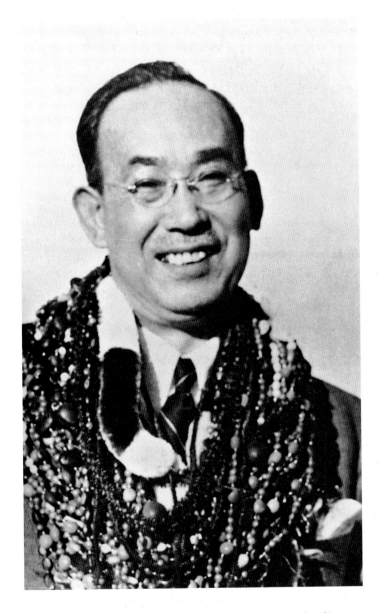

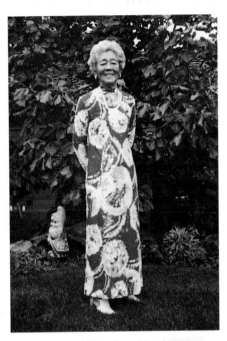

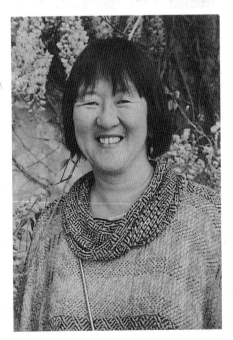

CLOCKWISE FROM ABOVE: Dr Chujiro Hayashi, Dr Usui's chosen successor; Hawayo Takata, the next Grand Master, who brought reiki to the USA, and Phyllis Lei Furumoto, the current Grand Master.

the five spiritual principles

Dr Usui created these five principles after working in the beggars' quarter in Kyoto, Japan where he realized his patients did not appreciate his free healing because they refused to take responsibility for their lives (see page 11). The principles are thoughts on appreciating life, and how to grow and change. Some believe they came from guidelines on living a fulfilled life by the Meiji Emperor of Japan (1868–1912), others that they originated from Dr Usui's Christian beliefs. The guidelines may vary with each reiki master and can be used as part of meditation.

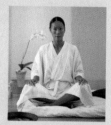

1 Just for today, do not worry

There is always a divine purpose to everything and when we worry we forget this. Worrying also means that we have lost faith and creates restrictions; it does not achieve anything, but wastes energy and causes tension and stress. Dr Usui was trying to remind people to trust that the Universe will always provide our needs if we give out clear messages. If you have a worry, let go of it today, ask for divine help and trust that the problem will be solved.

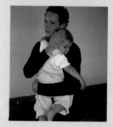

2 Just for today, do not anger

When our expectations about ourselves and other people are disappointed, or we don't satisfy our needs and desires we can become angry. Anger is necessary in the right situation as it can bring about change, but it is also destructive and we can hurt people by our outbursts. Getting angry is your own choice and often is just a habitual reaction to certain situations. Taking several deep breaths and responding more rationally or sympathetically when you feel this reaction can be very effective. Dr Usui did not expect people to avoid anger completely, but instead to try and respond to the cause with more positive feelings.

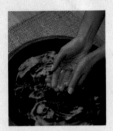

Earn your living honestly

This principle refers to all the work that we undertake, even simple everyday tasks such as cooking meals. You need to respect any job that you do and consider it to be satisfying and valuable, whether it is paid or voluntary work. When a person earns a living honestly they can trust in their own abilities to support themselves. It is also about being honest with yourself and others, and liking yourself. Dr Usui knew that dishonesty weighed heavily on many people, and that living a more honest life would lead them to be more in touch with their creative side as well as their life's purpose.

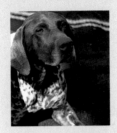

Show gratitude to all living things

Being grateful for everything that we have reinforces the abundance that is in our lives and encourages more to flow in. It works on the principle that "you get back what you give out". As your consciousness becomes connected spiritually to the Universal energy, you will realize that every living thing is part of you, and you are part of it. In this world there is no place for prejudice or hurting people. Everyone, including plants, animals, birds and insects, should be valued and given respect. Dr Usui knew that when people showed gratitude for these varied things, it encouraged joy, success and prosperity into their lives.

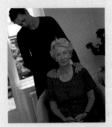

Honour your parents and elders

Our parents, who gave us life, should always be shown respect. Even if the relationship is not a happy one, respect can help to resolve some of the negative feelings. We learn from teachers of any age as well as our elders, so they too should be honoured. In fact, loving actions could be extended to every living thing. The inhumane actions of people to each other and the planet have had disastrous effects. And now many people accept that for our planet to survive and grow, we have got to become more positive. Start with loving actions to friends and family, and then try to extend it to everyone you meet.

the reiki symbols

Symbols have been part of many cultures, particularly eastern, for centuries. They are believed to have a unique power as they are thought to have so many different meanings that act on the mind, spirit and emotions. Many ancient symbols, some still in use today, were represented in art form and revered by ancient civilizations. In reiki, four special symbols are used: three that Dr Usui received on Mount Kuri Yami during his spiritual retreat are given to reiki students during their Second Degree initiation (see pages 18–21) and the fourth is taught exclusively to reiki masters. They are calligraphic symbols that are a very important part of the reiki healing system and are activated by special mantras which are taught to the students at the same time. The symbols help to make a stronger connection between the reiki healer and the life-force energy that they are channelling. They have to be learned and memorized after the attunement as no written record of them can be kept. Because of the sacred and deeply spiritual nature of the symbols and the fact that they are meant to be kept private and secret, they are not printed in this book.

unique to reiki

The symbols are a unique part of reiki and set it apart from other practical healing methods. They are thought to reveal parts of our inner selves that are hidden deep within us. Reiki is believed to use symbols because they contain a special power or energy that helps in the spiritual path, which is just as much a part of reiki as the physical healing. The three symbols taught at the Second Degree help in specific areas: one increases the reiki healing power that is first channelled at the First Degree initiation, helping to clear away any negative energies and give protection to the healer, another helps to heal mental and emotional problems and can also improve memory capacity and learning abilities. The last symbol is used for absent healing, to send to an unwell person anywhere in the world at any time. This type of healing can also be sent into the past (for emotional legacies) or to the future (as protection from worries to come). The fourth symbol is given solely to reiki masters to use during the attunement procedure to connect their students to the reiki healing energy.

becoming a healer –
the reiki initiations

You can use the healing positions shown in this book to some effect without being initiated, but reiki is a simple hands-on healing method to learn. Any adult or child can be attuned or initiated to the healing energy by a reiki master. To treat yourself or someone else you need to have the reiki initiations. These are divided into three degrees; at the Third Degree the initiant becomes a reiki master. Many people are happy to treat their family and friends with First Degree Reiki (Reiki I) and go no further, but if you want to continue with the training it is best to wait at least three months to get used to the energy before taking the Second Degree course. To continue to the Third Degree level to become a master it is advised that you leave a further year after the Second Degree. The reason that the attunements are done gradually is that the person being initiated would not be able to take the force of the energy they are receiving all at once. The physical and etheric (see pages 24–25) body needs to adjust gradually to the change in their vibratory level. Also the student needs to take time to absorb the reiki teachings.

Some reiki masters recommend that students build in a three-day period before training during which they eat light meals and avoid alcohol or recreational drugs to prepare their bodies for the energy. Attending a small training group with a maximum of 15 students with one master present is preferable to larger groups.

first degree reiki

Training for First Degree Reiki or Reiki I normally involves four sessions, with one attunement taking place per session. Often the training takes place over a weekend, but it can be held over four evenings. Every reiki master will include his or her own personal interpretation in the training, but the basic structure is the same.

The first day generally begins with everybody introducing themselves and giving their reasons for attending the course. The reiki master often then tells the story of how he or she came to reiki, explains the historical background and discusses the five spiritual principles behind the practical healing. The first attunement is given, with the second usually following after a break. The students can then feel the energy flowing through their hands and are taught the self-treatment positions (these can vary slightly between masters). The master also explains why they need to follow a 21–30-day cleansing period where they perform a full treatment on themselves daily. The minimum of 21 days mirrors the time that Dr Usui spent fasting, but it is also the time that it takes for the energy to move through the chakras. This cleansing detoxifies the body and as a result, can induce mild sickness or diarrhoea. It may cause physical changes in the body and balance the mind and emotions. Daily self-treatment enables the students to heal themselves emotionally and physically before treating others as well as helping them to become aware of how the energy flows.

On the second day people often recount their experiences of the previous day before the third and fourth attunements take place. The last attunement helps to ground the energy they have received and gets rid of the slightly "spacey", light-headed feeling that students often experience.

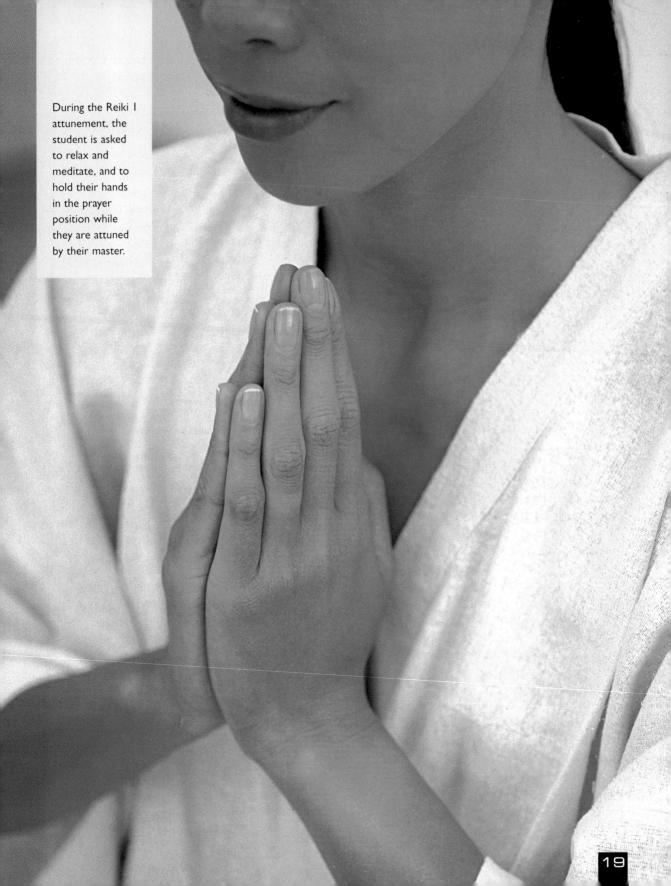

During the Reiki I attunement, the student is asked to relax and meditate, and to hold their hands in the prayer position while they are attuned by their master.

Students may also be told how they can use reiki for their personal and spiritual growth, or how it can treat pets or plants, for example. The rest of the day is spent with the students learning the positions to treat others. They may also be taught how to help someone through an emotional healing crisis. Any questions that come up will normally be answered throughout the day. The session often ends with all the students giving and receiving a full treatment. These First Degree initiations are believed to open the heart, hand and crown chakras and the energy flow can often dramatically affect these areas. Reiki is an oral tradition but sometimes basic handouts showing the hand positions are given out.

second degree reiki

Many people are happy to stay at the First Degree Reiki level but others will want to have a deeper involvement and decide to do the Second Degree (Reiki II). This is also the level that is recommended for people who want to become reiki practitioners. The course is often split into three sessions, held over a weekend or three evenings. This stage needs more commitment because the attunement that is received particularly works on the student's etheric body (see pages 24–25) affecting them mentally and emotionally, and increasing their intuitive abilities. Again a 21- or 30-day cleansing period is recommended after the course to assist with the integration of the energy.

At this level the students are given the ability to channel much more energy than at the First Degree. Only one attunement is given which opens up the chakras more fully. The master then shows them how to use the three symbols and mantras (these need to be learned by heart) that activate them (see pages 16–17). This process intensifies the reiki energy and gives the students the ability to do absent (distant) healing using the symbols. All that is needed is a name or a picture of a person so that they can connect with them before sending the energy.

This energy can also be sent to the past to heal negative patterns or to the future, for luck.

third degree reiki

This level of reiki (Reiki III) trains the student to be a master and teacher. When the Reiki Alliance was formed in 1981, the Masters decided that those who wished to teach the Usui system needed to be an apprentice to a reiki master for at least 12 months. In the 1970s, Mrs Takata had already set the Master's fee at $10,000, a considerable amount at this time. This high fee, which remains roughly the same today, was set to reflect the commitment needed for this specialized training.

During the apprentice year the student learns amongst other things to develop his or her personality to gain the maturity and spiritual understanding to teach others. He is given a further symbol and mantra, and one more attunement which substantially increases his ability to channel the reiki energy. Learning how to organize reiki classes and teach reiki students is also included in the training. Becoming a reiki master commits the student to reiki for life and because of the spiritual changes that come about, other aspects of their life, such as relationships or lifestyle, can be affected.

Some independent masters are now teaching Third Degree Reiki as a course rather than an apprenticeship and the charges are much lower. The course is also sometimes split into two levels: reiki master (or master practitioner) and reiki master/teacher. Often an additional attunement, extra symbols and mantras for other healing traditions are included. A short course is not always the easiest route and each person must make a decision about the training needed. A reiki master must have a good understanding of the Usui tradition and be committed to help others to achieve their full potential, both physically and spiritually.

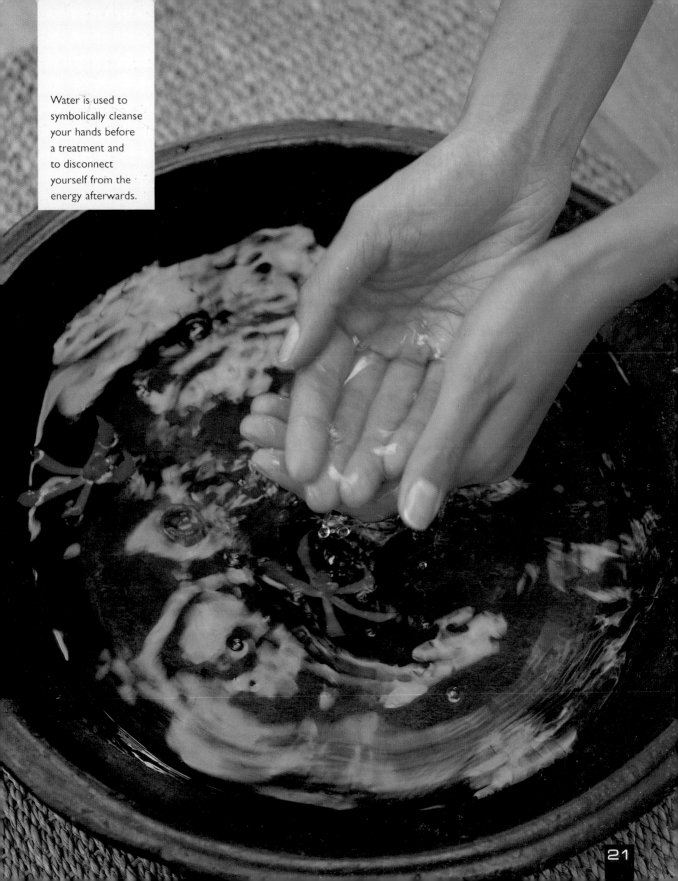

Water is used to
symbolically cleanse
your hands before
a treatment and
to disconnect
yourself from the
energy afterwards.

the endocrine system

When a reiki treatment is given the healing energy goes of its own accord where it is needed in the body. So, if a person was suffering from a pain in one of their legs, the healer would give a full treatment and spend extra time on the painful leg, but there would be no guarantee that the pain would be immediately cured as the energy would first go to the place where it was most needed, which may not be where the pain is manifesting itself. This is why several hour-long treatments will normally be required for someone to feel improvement in a painful condition.

the function of the endocrine system

This system is part of the orthodox Western school of medicine and consists of seven glands: the pituitary, pineal, thyroid and parathyroids, the thymus, the islets of Langerhans in the pancreas, the adrenals and the gonads (men) and ovaries (women).

The endocrine glands release chemicals known as hormones into the bloodstream and circulatory system to stimulate or modify the action of the organs and tissues. The hormones help the body to react to hunger, disease and infection, and prepare it for physical movement, stress or reproduction. They are also involved in metabolism, growth, ageing and maintaining inner stability, known as homeostasis. All the glands in the endocrine system work independently of each other, but if one is underactive or overactive it affects all of them.

When hand positions are used on the head the energy affects the pituitary and pineal glands. The pituitary gland coordinates the other glands and regulates sleep, body fluids and stimulates growth. The pineal gland controls sexual development and skin pigmentation. When the hands are placed on the throat area the thyroid and parathyroid glands are influenced. These glands control metabolism and help balance levels of calcium and phosphorous essential for the healthy functioning of bones, nerves and muscles. As the hands move over the heart area the thymus gland is affected. The thymus helps to promote a healthy immune system, producing "T" cells which protect the body against disease.

When the hands are placed on the upper abdomen the islets of Langerhans in the pancreas and the adrenal glands receive the energy. The islets of Langerhans in the pancreas secrete insulin and glucogen, maintaining glucose levels in the blood. The adrenal glands sit above the kidneys and the outer layer of glands control the levels of salt, water and sugar in the body and influence secondary sexual characteristics (the physical features that appear at puberty). The inner layer releases adrenaline, the hormone necessary for the stress "fight or flight" reaction. When the hands work on the reproductive glands, the gonads or ovaries are affected. These glands regulate fertility and help control our emotions.

the two systems

The aim of using the hand positions in a full-body reiki treatment is to create balance and harmony in the endocrine system and the chakras, the Eastern diagnostic system. In reiki and other healing methods these two systems are believed to be intrinsically linked. The glands release hormones which affect our physical health, but when reiki is given, the chakras – our spiritual centres of emotional wellbeing – are also affected. The adrenal glands, despite being higher up the body than the reproductive organs, are linked to the root chakra because when this area is treated with reiki, it swiftly flows up the spinal cord to the adrenals.

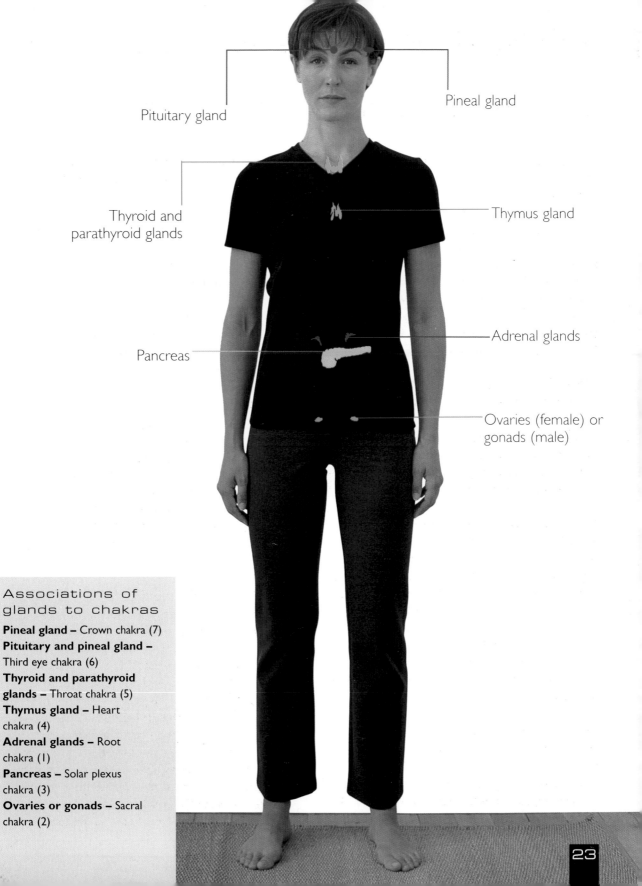

Pituitary gland

Pineal gland

Thyroid and
parathyroid glands

Thymus gland

Adrenal glands

Pancreas

Ovaries (female) or
gonads (male)

Associations of glands to chakras

Pineal gland – Crown chakra (7)

Pituitary and pineal gland –
Third eye chakra (6)

**Thyroid and parathyroid
glands –** Throat chakra (5)

Thymus gland – Heart
chakra (4)

Adrenal glands – Root
chakra (1)

Pancreas – Solar plexus
chakra (3)

Ovaries or gonads – Sacral
chakra (2)

the seven chakras

The chakras are spiritual energy centres that are located in seven major points on the etheric body (aura) which surrounds the physical body. The first is situated at the base of the spine, with the seventh being at the top of the body on the crown of the head. Chakra is a Sanskrit work meaning wheel, and people who are clairvoyant often say that they can see the chakras as spinning wheels. The chakras are emotional centres linked to the physical body through the endocrine glands and organs that are situated in the same area of the body (see page 22–23). The endocrine system controls the hormones in the body, which in turn greatly affect people's moods and emotions.

The chakras can react to light energy which causes them to vibrate at a certain frequency that relates to a sound and specific colour. The energy that flows through the chakras can become disrupted due to emotional upset or stress in the mind. If this is not resolved, it can eventually lead to physical illness. When a chakra is not functioning well, the speed at which it spins is seen to either slow down or speed up. This will also relate to malfunctioning in the related organ or gland. The chakras can be influenced by colours that you are wearing – orange, for example, would affect the sacral chakra. They can also be balanced by a reiki treatment. In fact, when the hands are placed on the body they are right over the seven main chakras. If one chakra is out of balance it dramatically affects the functioning of the other ones, so it is better to give a full treatment to restore harmony. As more treatments are given it will become easier to sense any imbalances in the "invisible" chakra areas.

Name	Function	Colour
First, the root chakra	Governs survival and power. Illness can manifest as bone or reproductive problems.	red
Second, the sacral chakra	Controls creativity and sexuality. Problems may manifest in sexual issues.	orange
Third, the solar plexus chakra	Relates to intellect and personal power. Blockages are linked to mental upsets or stomach problems.	yellow
Fourth, the heart chakra	The emotional centre, it relates to love and relationship issues. Upset in this area can reduce your capacity to offer and receive love and affection.	green
Fifth, the throat chakra	This area controls metabolism and relates to communication. Imbalance or blockages can make you want to control others, and may manifest as throat disorders.	turquoise blue
Sixth, the third eye chakra	This is where our intuitive powers and clairvoyant abilities come from. Blockages can be associated with headaches or eye problems.	indigo
Seventh, the crown chakra	The spiritual centre which helps us to love and appreciate beautiful objects and art. Problems here can be linked with feelings of isolation and despair.	purple

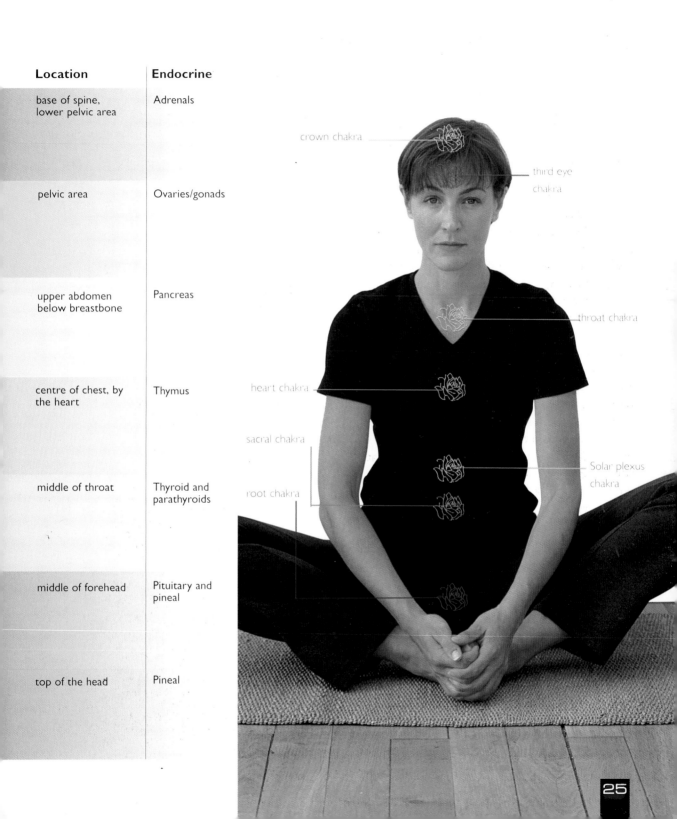

Location	Endocrine
base of spine, lower pelvic area	Adrenals
pelvic area	Ovaries/gonads
upper abdomen below breastbone	Pancreas
centre of chest, by the heart	Thymus
middle of throat	Thyroid and parathyroids
middle of forehead	Pituitary and pineal
top of the head	Pineal

crown chakra

third eye chakra

throat chakra

heart chakra

sacral chakra

Solar plexus chakra

root chakra

listening to your body

emotional patterns that become physical

An illness or ailment will normally happen because there is a blockage in one of the chakras (spiritual energy centres). The mind is very powerful and can positively or negatively affect our physical health and wellbeing. So sometimes, if we are not willing to acknowledge an emotional upset, our body will then show it as a physical discomfort. This chart is by no means a comprehensive list of all the illnesses and the chakras they affect, but it is a means of looking at ourselves and other people to see what is the probable emotional cause of the existing or past ailment. By using reiki on ourselves and others, we can heal any damaging energy blockages and give ourselves a more positive outlook on life, encouraging a balanced and healthy mind, body and spirit.

Ailment	Likely emotional cause
root chakra (base of spine)	
Athlete's foot	Frustration at not being accepted, not moving forward easily.
Leg problems	A fear of moving on in life. Problems with the upper legs can be often connected with childhood upsets which won't let you progress. Trouble with the thighs can be connected with trusting yourself.
Knee problems	These can be associated with fear, a stubborn pride and ego and inflexibility.
Fat on thighs	Anger from childhood, often directed at the father.
Fat on hips	Stubborn anger that is directed at the parents.
Hip problems	A fear of resolving major decisions; worries about being unloved, or feelings of resentment and guilt.
Lower back pain	Worries about money and lack of financial support.
Kidney problems	Disappointment or failure in life, self-criticism. This area stores annoyed feelings and anger, so when kidney problems arise it may indicate that these emotions have not been resolved.
sacral chakra (pelvic area)	
Middle back problems	Wanting people to leave you alone; feelings of guilt.
Fat on stomach	Anger at being denied proper emotional nourishment.
Constipation	A refusal to let go of the past or old ideas, or a fear of authority.
Diarrhoea	Fear and rejection of anything that may be beneficial to you.
Bladder problems	Anxiety, holding onto old ideas. A fear of releasing the past.
Thrush	Associated with angry feelings over making the wrong decisions.

Ailment	Likely emotional cause
solar plexus chakra (upper abdomen area)	
Abdominal cramp	A fear, which makes you reluctant to get on in life.
Belching	A fear that there will not be enough, so you gulp down life too quickly.
Gastritis	A prolonged feeling of uncertainty and a sense that all is not well.
Indigestion	A fear and dread in the gut, overwhelming anxiety.
Nausea	Can be linked to a fear of life, rejecting an idea or experience.
Stomach problems	A fear and dread of taking on anything new in life.
Gallstones	Bitter or hard feelings that can be condemning to other people.
heart chakra (centre of chest)	
Upper back pain	Linked to a lack of emotional support, a feeling that no one cares.
Middle back pain	A feeling of being burdened, wanting to get people off your back. Guilt.
Anxiety	Not trusting the flow of life and how it should proceed.
Lung problems	Breathing problems can represent a fear of taking in life. Can be related to depression or grief.
Heartburn	Too much fear, and a feeling that it is clutching at your heart.
throat chakra (middle of throat)	
Sore throat	Unable to express yourself, holding in feelings of anger.
Bad breath	Angry feelings and thoughts of revenge. Your experiences are stale and blocked.
Neck problems	Stubbornness and inflexibility have literally given you a pain in the neck.
Hay fever	Emotional congestion and feelings of guilt and persecution.
Tonsillitis	Fear and repressed emotions, no trust in other people.

Flu	A response to a lot of negative beliefs and fear.
Hyperthyroidism (overactive thyroid)	A feeling of rage at being left out of things.
Hypothyroidism (underactive thyroid)	Wanting to give up, feelings of being stifled.
Teeth problems	Indecisiveness over a long period. Inability to analyze ideas or to decide what to do.
Nose problems	Suffering from a stuffy nose can be connected with not recognizing your self-worth. A runny nose is linked with the need to ask for help and inner crying.
Headaches and migraines	Constantly criticizing yourself, fear of life, can also incorporate sexual fears.

third eye chakra (middle of forehead)

Dizziness	Feelings of wanting to take flight and run away, a refusal to look ahead.
Eyes – far sighted	A fear of things happening in the present.
Eyes – near sighted	A fear of what will happen in the future.
Earache	Anger held within. Not wanting to hear what is going on around you, or listening to your inner guidance.

crown chakra (top of the head)

Fainting	Feeling that you can't cope with life, so you literally shut down.
Neuralgia	Feelings of anguish and guilt over communication problems.

preparing for reiki

When you start to give treatments to friends and family and other people after receiving First Degree Reiki training, you will need to set aside a suitable area in your home. If you want to work as a reiki healer at a natural health centre or from home it is normally advised that you wait until you have done the Second Degree level. As a healer you will also need to have professional indemnity insurance and public liability cover. The fees that you can charge normally equate to the cost of a massage treatment.

The area that you use for reiki treatments, be it a bedroom, or part of your living area needs to be well aired, clean and tidy with a warm and relaxed atmosphere. You can cleanse the room with reiki before you start by just sitting quietly and letting the energy flow out through your hands and concentrating on clearing any negativity. Ideally, you should have a massage table set at the right height for you to sit comfortably or stand at and which allows you to work around the person you are treating. Alternatively, cover a strong, rectangular dining or kitchen table with a duvet, use a firm bed or a duvet on the floor, but bear in mind that squatting on the floor for an hour can be uncomfortable.

Although the person remains fully clothed (you should, however, ask them to remove their shoes) when lying down during treatment, they may become a bit cold during the hour-long session so it is a good idea to have a light blanket to cover them. You will also need a pillow for their head and possibly under their knees. Incense can be burned in the room before treatment begins, but if the person suffers from breathing disorders try using a calming essential oil such as lavender, diluted in water, in an oil burner. A lit candle plus some soothing, gentle music in the background can help to create the right atmosphere.

When the person arrives for the treatment it is a good idea to have a brief chat. You do not need to take a medical history, and if they are a friend or a member of your family, you will probably already know their problems. Discuss why they want a treatment and whether they are seeking relief from a physical or emotional problem. This is called setting an intent, and you should do this before treating yourself as well as others to decide where the energy needs to go. Note down any drugs they are taking and any other complementary therapies they have tried. Have a clock nearby that you can easily read, so that you can time yourself during the hour-long treatment in the different positions.

getting ready

■ Turn your answerphone on or turn down the ringer on your telephone and switch off any mobile phones. Try to ensure that you are not interrupted by children or pets.

■ Remove your watch and any other jewellery before you start and ask the person you are treating if they mind doing the same.

■ Wash your hands before you begin and again at the end of the session to disconnect yourself from the recipient's energy.

■ Try not to eat any very spicy or garlic-flavoured food before treatments as the smell can be irritating.

■ Strong perfume or aftershave can also be an unwelcome distraction.

■ Relax yourself or meditate for a short time before a healing session to clear your mind of busy thoughts.

■ Keep a box of tissues handy in case strong emotions are released during treatment.

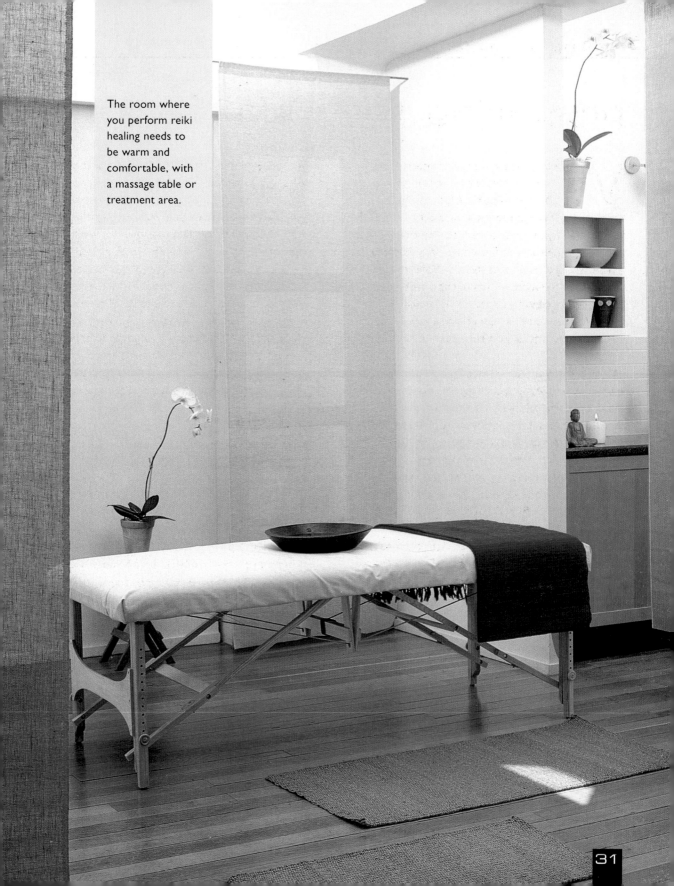

The room where you perform reiki healing needs to be warm and comfortable, with a massage table or treatment area.

the reiki treatment

Discuss what happens during a treatment, explaining how the energy is channelled through you, and that the healing energy may be experienced as a warm, cold or a tingling sensation. Mention that the person being treated may become aware of a sensation in the area of an old wound when the healing affects that area, or that they may find themselves crying as an emotional blockage is released. Explain the 12 hand positions saying how they start at the head (see page 36), and are held for about 5 minutes (3 after Second Degree Reiki), and tell them how they will start the treatment lying on their backs and then turn over onto their stomachs for the last four. Whether you allow talking or questions during treatment is an individual decision, but often you will find that the person being treated will soon drift off into a light sleep.

After treatment make sure that you both drink a glass of water to flush out the toxins that have been released. You should also wash your hands to disconnect from the energy. Advise the person treated to drink more water over the next 24–48 hours to help detoxification, and avoid alcohol during this period as it can cause unpleasant aftereffects.

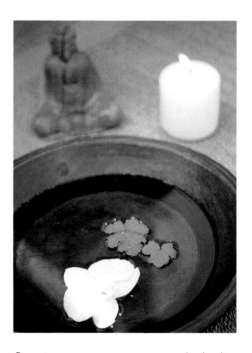

Reactions to treatment vary as the healing energy goes where it is needed, and both the healer and recipient are affected. Creative ideas or solutions to problems can surface or, more painfully, old emotions or anger can be released. People can have flu-like symptoms or suffer aches and pains in old injury areas. Sometimes, as toxins are released, more frequent bladder or bowel movements are experienced. These symptoms can be more severe after a first treatment as the purification process takes place. A far more pleasant reaction is the deep relaxation and a feeling of being at peace that people often experience. Reiki is suitable for pregnant women and their babies and will help to alleviate morning sickness and lower back pain.

self-treatment

■ When you are treating yourself, make sure that you are lying or sitting on a comfortable, padded surface, such as a bed or large cushion. Untrained people can also follow the self-treatment positions, but will need reiki training to get the full benefit from them as the attunements give the extra flow of energy. Again each of the 12 positions should be held for 5 minutes (3 minutes at Second Degree Reiki).

If a person is feeling very relaxed and slightly "spacey" after treatment you may need to "ground" them by sitting them down for a while before they leave, especially if they are driving.

safety tips

■ Treating someone with a pacemaker or similar mechanized device is not recommended as the effects of the reiki energy on them are unknown.

■ Reiki can help to heal broken bones, but treatment should not be given until the bone has been set in plaster as it might make it knit at the wrong angle.

■ Always warn clients that have diabetes to check their insulin level carefully immediately after a treatment as the reiki can affect it.

■ Babies and children do not need such a long treatment as adults, in fact, 20–30 minutes is normally sufficient.

■ Treatment should not be given or received after drinking alcohol as it can distort the reiki energy and may bring about some unpleasant reactions.

■ Do not attempt to treat someone in a hospital if they have just had an anaesthetic prior to an operation.

■ It is better to give a reiki treatment to someone before or after a chemotherapy course, rather then during it, as it tends to reduce toxic levels. However, it is safe to give reiki to someone undergoing a radiotherapy course.

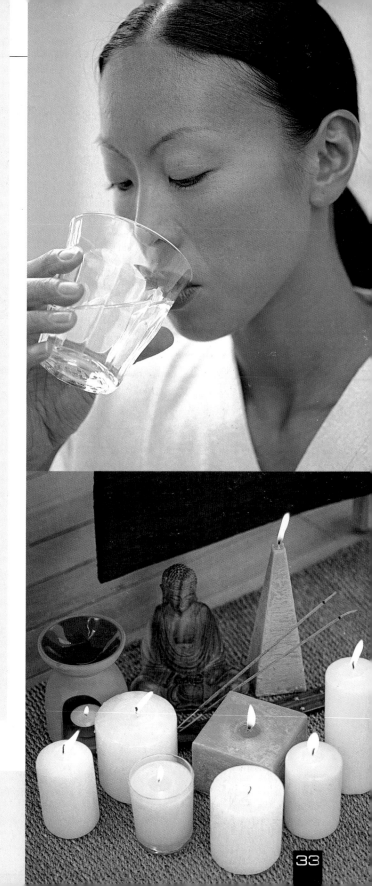

ABOVE RIGHT: A glass of water after a reiki treatment will help the detoxification process.
RIGHT: Candles can help create a calming atmosphere.

the twelve basic positions

Twelve hand positions are used by a healer in a hour-long reiki treatment and there are extra positions for treating the knees and feet (for treating others only). As a rule, you should hold each position for about 5 minutes, and when treating the head positions, try to turn your head to one side to avoid breathing on the recipient. Relax your hands, keeping your fingers and thumbs together and rest the heels of your hand lightly on their forehead, arching your fingers over their eyes and making sure they can breathe easily. The reiki treatment is most effective when you actually touch the person and you should try not to lose contact with their body throughout the treatment to avoid interrupting the flow of reiki energy. If, however, the recipient would prefer to avoid body contact, for example on their face, you can position your hands slightly above the face and the energy will still flow through.

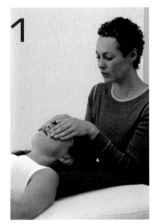

the front of the head

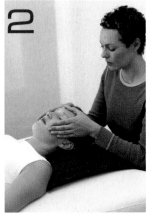

the temples

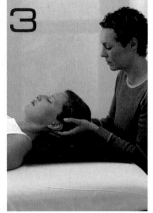

the back of the head

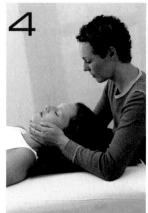

the throat and jaw

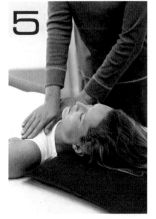

the heart

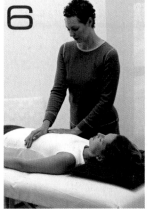

the ribcage

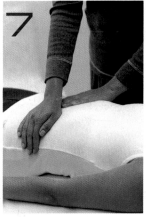

the abdomen

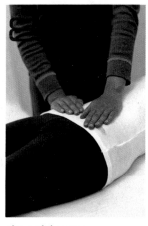

the pelvic area

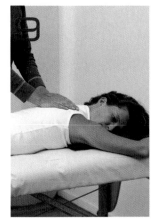

the shoulders

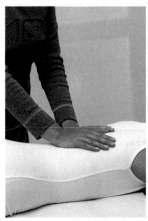

the shoulder blades

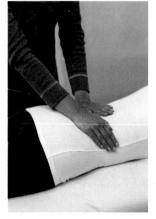

the lower back

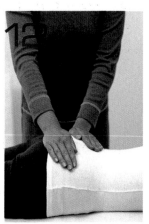

the tail bone

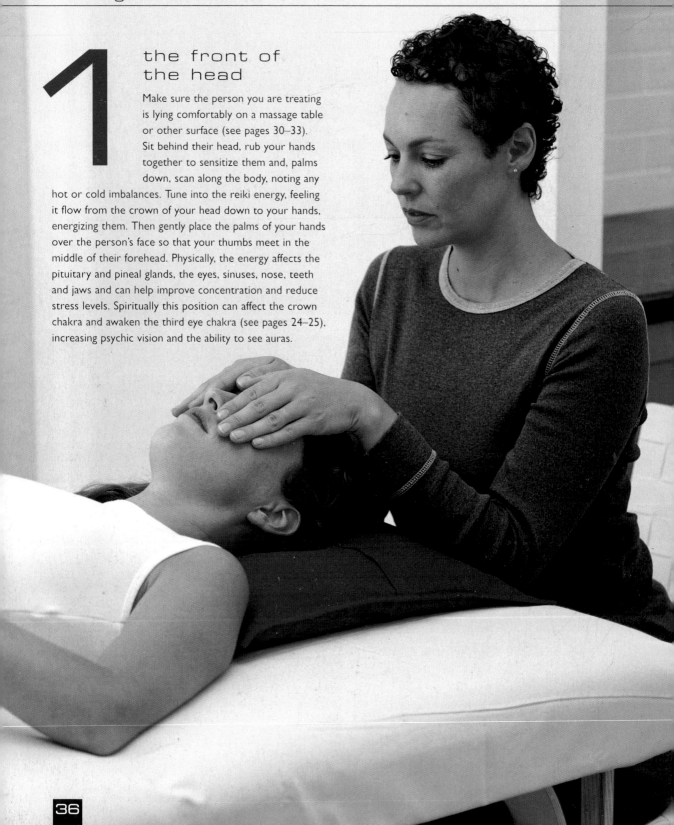

1 the front of the head

Make sure the person you are treating is lying comfortably on a massage table or other surface (see pages 30–33). Sit behind their head, rub your hands together to sensitize them and, palms down, scan along the body, noting any hot or cold imbalances. Tune into the reiki energy, feeling it flow from the crown of your head down to your hands, energizing them. Then gently place the palms of your hands over the person's face so that your thumbs meet in the middle of their forehead. Physically, the energy affects the pituitary and pineal glands, the eyes, sinuses, nose, teeth and jaws and can help improve concentration and reduce stress levels. Spiritually this position can affect the crown chakra and awaken the third eye chakra (see pages 24–25), increasing psychic vision and the ability to see auras.

self-treatment

Working on your head

Lie down on a bed or sit on a padded surface or chair and relax by breathing in and out deeply. Cup your hands slightly and place them, palms down, over your eyes. To treat the top of your head, move your hands up so that your palms are over your eyes. Experiment with the pressure of your hands until they feel comfortable. Visualize the energy moving down from the crown of your head energizing them; you may feel a sensation of heat in your hands, which will diminish when your body has absorbed what it needs. The energy affects or helps the areas or conditions described on page 36 and can also increase clarity of thought, improve your decision making, and increase your intuitive and inspirational abilities in the third eye chakra (see pages 24–25).

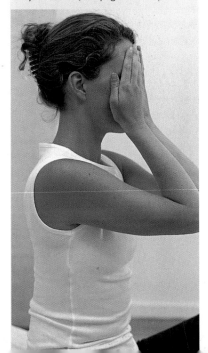

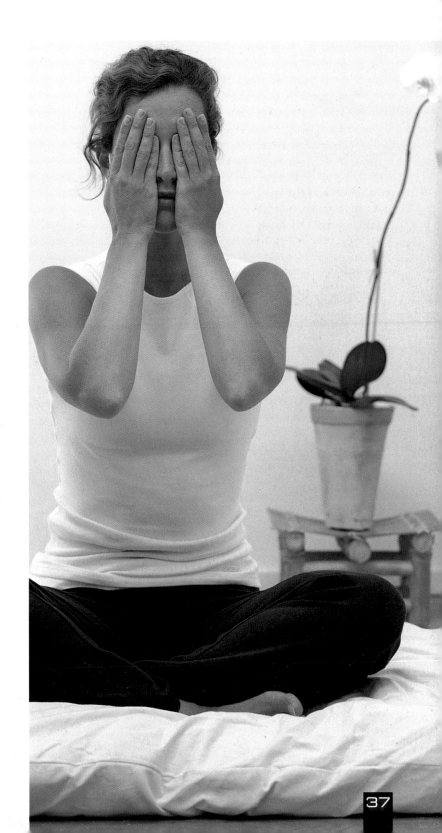

2 the temples

For the second position, without taking your hands off the person's body, slowly move them so that your palms are over the person's temples with your hands resting just above their ears. Your thumbs should meet in the middle of their forehead over the third eye chakra. In this position, the healing energy physically influences and helps to integrate the right and left parts of the brain and the eye muscles. It can also help relieve colds, headaches and motion sickness, and as with the first position, the pituitary and pineal glands will benefit from the energy. Emotionally, worry, shock and stress can be alleviated, and spiritually there may be an improvement in recalling dreams or past life. Mentally it can induce feelings of calm and increase memory retention.

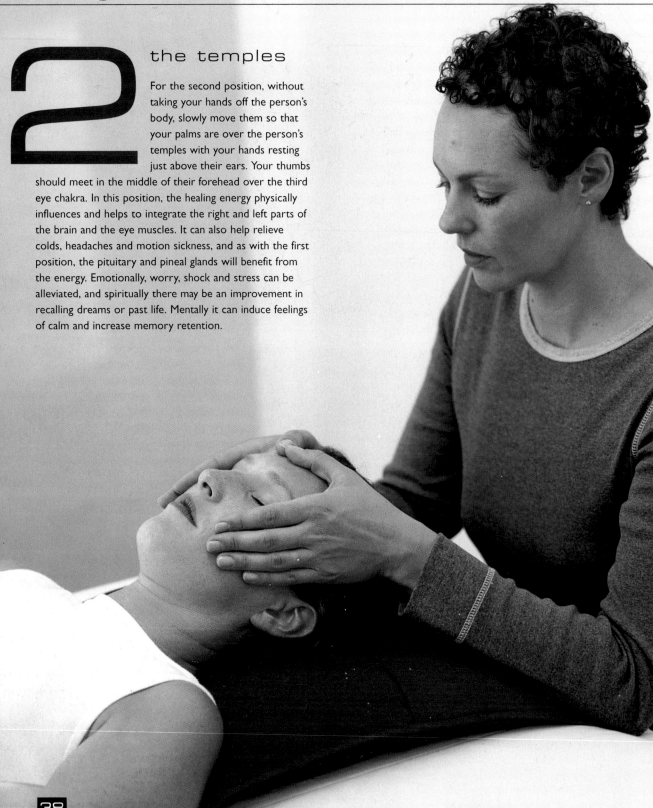

self-treatment

Working on your temples

Without taking your hands off your body, move your hands to the side of your head, just over the ears, so that you are covering your temples. You will begin to relax as the reiki energy flows into this area. The same areas and conditions will be affected or helped as mentioned on page 38. You may also experience a release of pent-up mental tension and an increase in your productive or creative abilities.

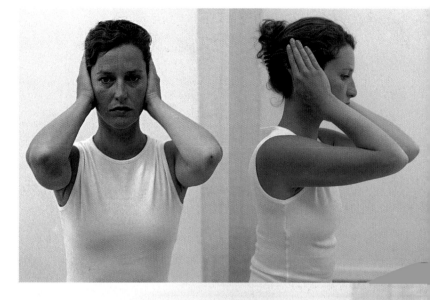

Working on the crown of your head

You can also try this alternative position which affects the same areas and ailments mentioned above. Move your hands from your face and, without losing contact with your body, place them palms down on the crown of your head with your fingers meeting in the middle. The crown chakra (see pages 24–25), which is thought to be the link to everyone's Higher Self (the all-knowing part of ourselves) is also stimulated by this position.

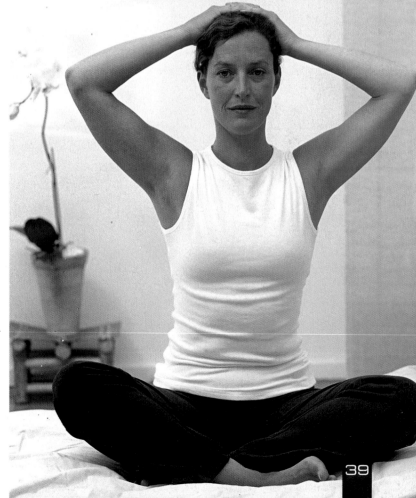

39

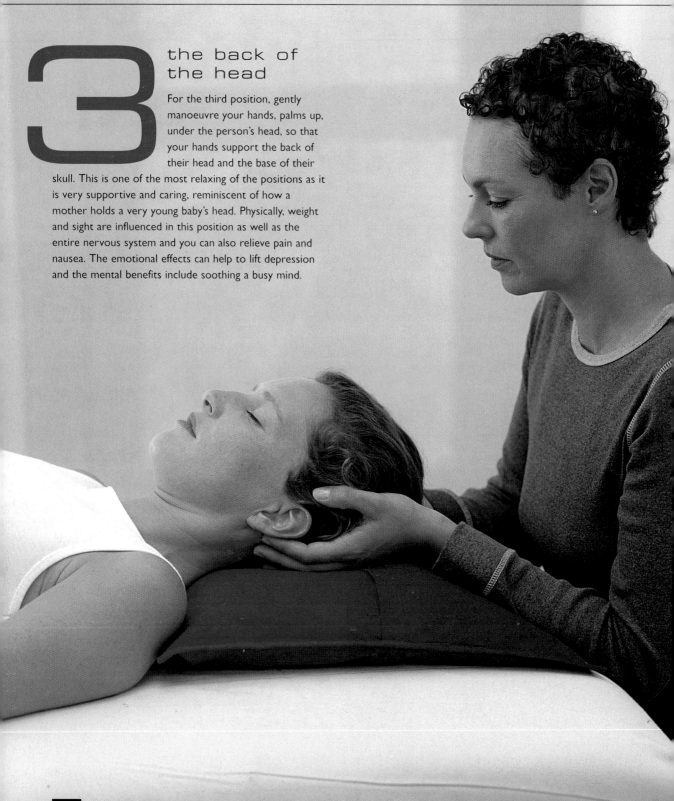

3 the back of the head

For the third position, gently manoeuvre your hands, palms up, under the person's head, so that your hands support the back of their head and the base of their skull. This is one of the most relaxing of the positions as it is very supportive and caring, reminiscent of how a mother holds a very young baby's head. Physically, weight and sight are influenced in this position as well as the entire nervous system and you can also relieve pain and nausea. The emotional effects can help to lift depression and the mental benefits include soothing a busy mind.

self-treatment

Working on the base of your head

Move your hands from the temples to the back of your head and clasp them one on top of the other on the base of your skull over the occipital lobe as shown right. The same areas and conditions will be affected or helped as detailed on page 40. This caring position will also help with relaxation. It affects our will, which if it is restricted, can make us undervalue ourselves and give away power to other people.

Working on the back of your head

You can also try this alternative position (shown below), which affects the same areas and conditions described above, if you find it easier to hold. Place your hands, palms down, one above the other on the back of your head. The body also absorbs a lot of energy in this area, and a well-balanced, harmonized body will help you perform well.

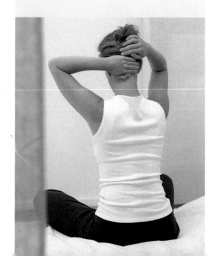

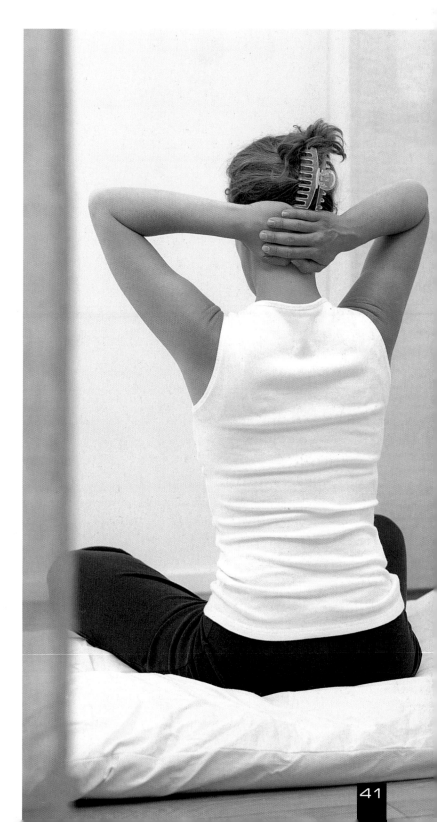

4

the throat and jaw

For the fourth position, move your hands to the person's throat, cupping your palms over the bottom of their jawline and throat. The energy affects the tonsils, throat, larynx and thyroid and parathryoid glands and can help to balance high or low blood pressure and increase lymphatic drainage. Metabolic and weight problems and anorexia may also be improved. The jaw is a place where much emotion is stored, so working on this area can remove feelings of resentment, animosity or anger.

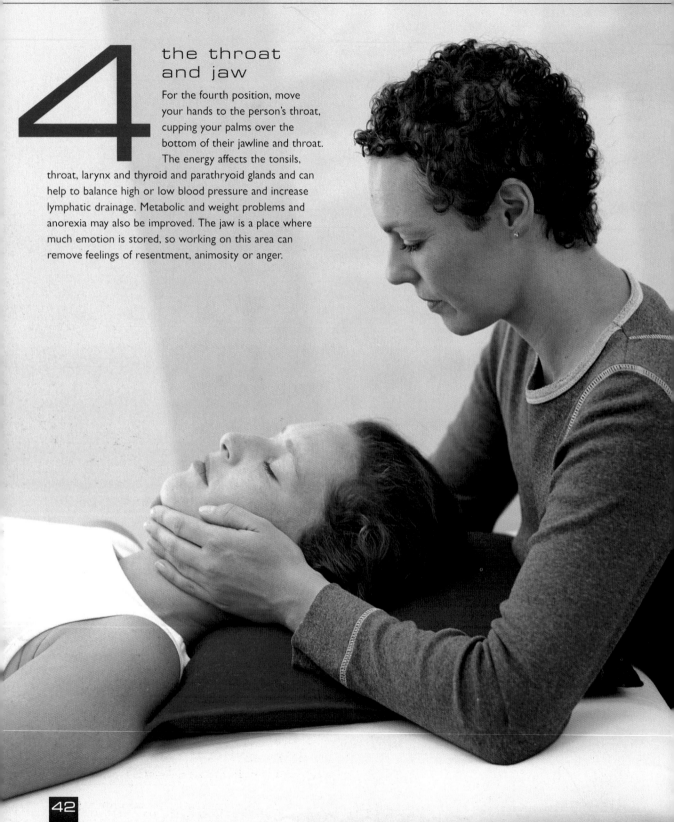

self-treatment

Working on your throat and jaw

For this final head position (shown right), place your hands around your throat so that you are holding the bottom of your jawline, bringing the heels of your hands together under your chin. The same areas and conditions will be affected or helped as mentioned on page 42. Mentally, the energy can help to calm you and allow you to think more clearly. Emotionally, it can make you feel more confident and joyful.

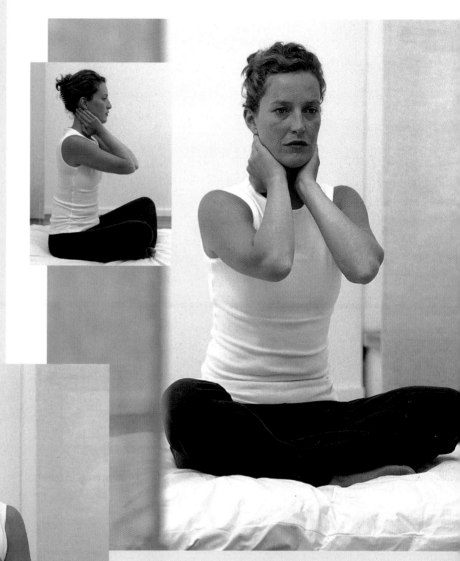

Working on your throat area

You can also use this alternative position (left) to treat this area. Place one hand on your throat and then put your other hand directly underneath it on your chest. This position will also affect the same areas and ailments mentioned on these pages. The throat chakra (see pages 24–25) is also stimulated, which can often feel like pins and needles, or you may want to clear your throat or cough. These sensations are a good sign as it normally means that a blockage representing something you meant to say or had been holding back has been shifted. You will now find it easier to express what you truly feel.

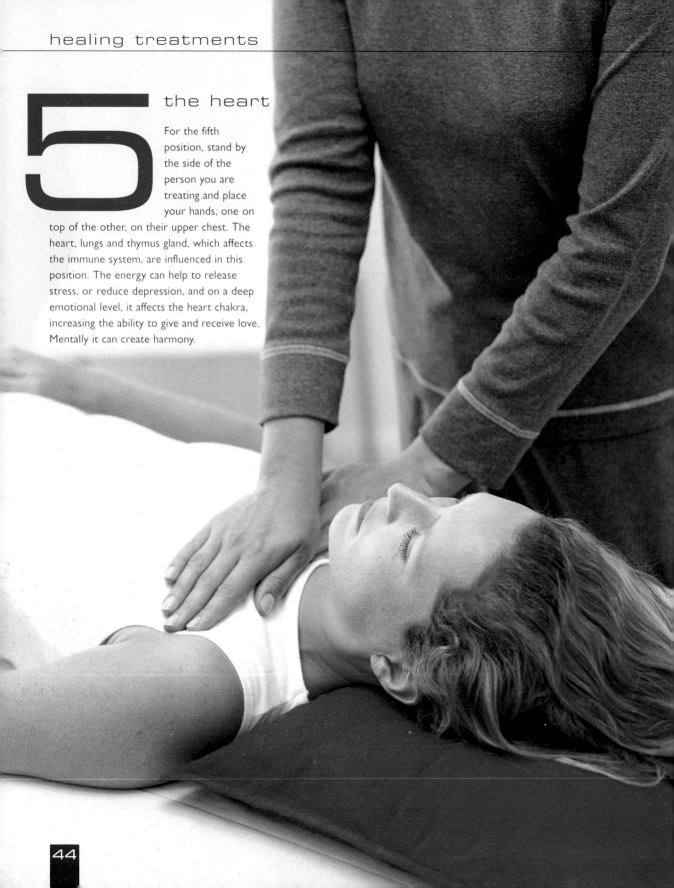

5 the heart

For the fifth position, stand by the side of the person you are treating and place your hands, one on top of the other, on their upper chest. The heart, lungs and thymus gland, which affects the immune system, are influenced in this position. The energy can help to release stress, or reduce depression, and on a deep emotional level, it affects the heart chakra, increasing the ability to give and receive love. Mentally it can create harmony.

self-treatment

Working on your heart
Move your hands to your chest area, placing them on either side of your chest bone as shown on the right. The same areas and conditions will be affected as detailed left. This is one of our most sensitive areas and many of us build barriers around our heart chakra to protect ourselves from being hurt (see pages 24–25). These barriers can be slowly broken down by the reiki energy. Sometimes you can sense a physical movement in this area, perhaps a tingling sensation or gentle tremors, or you may feel the blood flow increase as this process begins. Removing these blockages will really help you to get to know your emotional side.

Working on your heart area
An alternative position to try is to place one hand on top of the other in the centre of your chest (shown below). Again the energy works on the same areas and conditions as detailed previously. Working on this area will make you more willing to risk becoming vulnerable by giving love to someone.

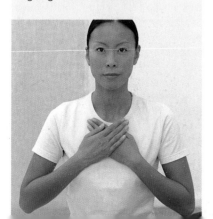

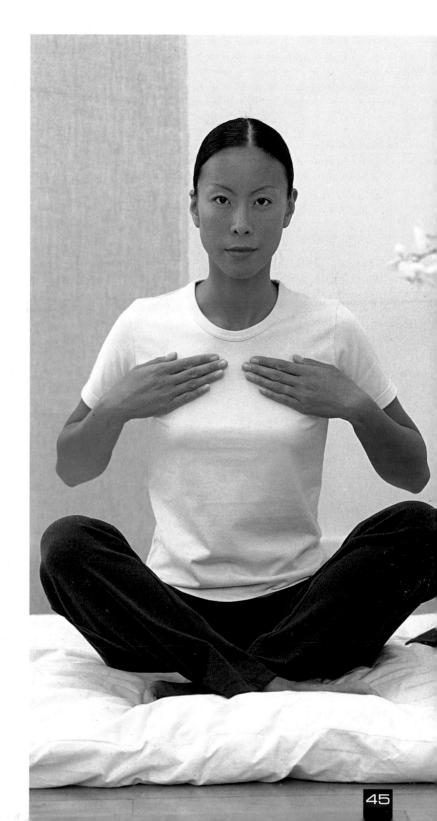

6 the rib cage

For the sixth position, move your hands down the side of the body and place them one in front of the other on their ribcage and over their solar plexus, just below their chest. The reiki energy working in this area will affect the stomach, spleen, liver, gall bladder and digestion. It can particularly alleviate any stomach upsets and can help to release body toxins from the spleen and liver. Emotionally, it can help release any hidden fears and assist relaxation, while mentally it can help to "centre" or balance both the physical and mental state of the person being treated.

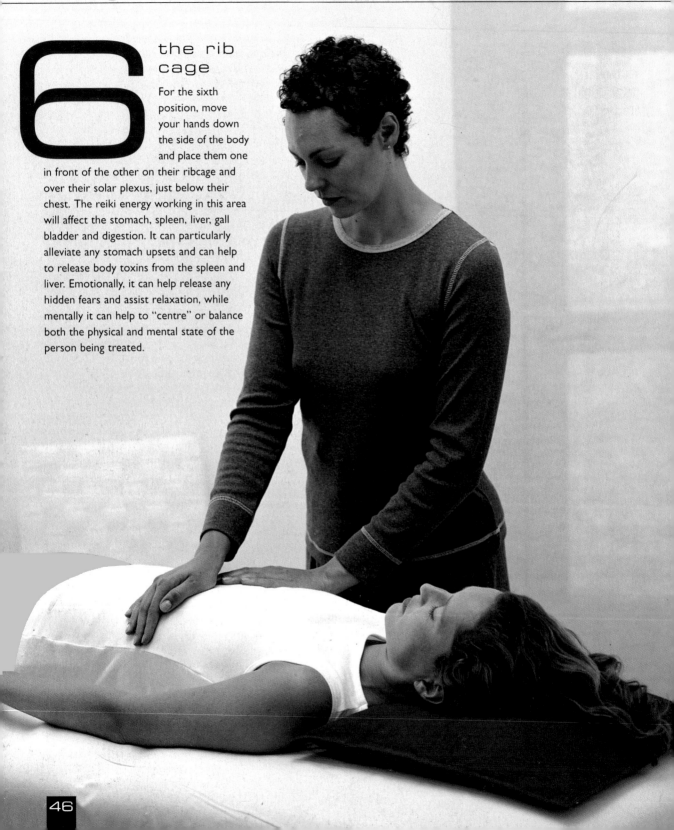

self-treatment

Working on your ribcage

Slowly move your hands down from your chest to rest on each side of your ribcage over the solar plexus, ensuring that your fingers meet in the middle. Sending the energy here will affect the same areas and conditions as mentioned on page 46. It will also help to balance the solar plexus chakra (see pages 24–25), which is considered to be our position of power in the body. When you are hurt emotionally, it often feels as if someone has punched you in the stomach. This may leave you feeling defenceless and hesitant, unprotected and lacking in self-confidence. Harmonizing this area will make you feel more secure and sure of yourself, and enable you to move on easily so that you can make some real progress in your life.

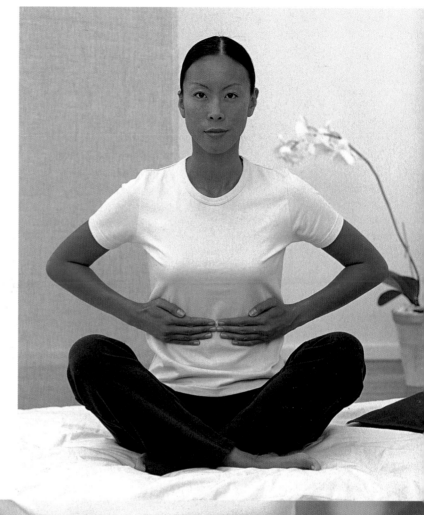

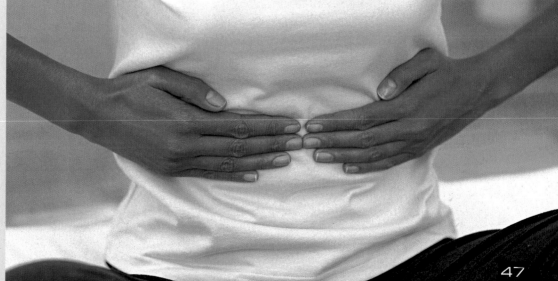

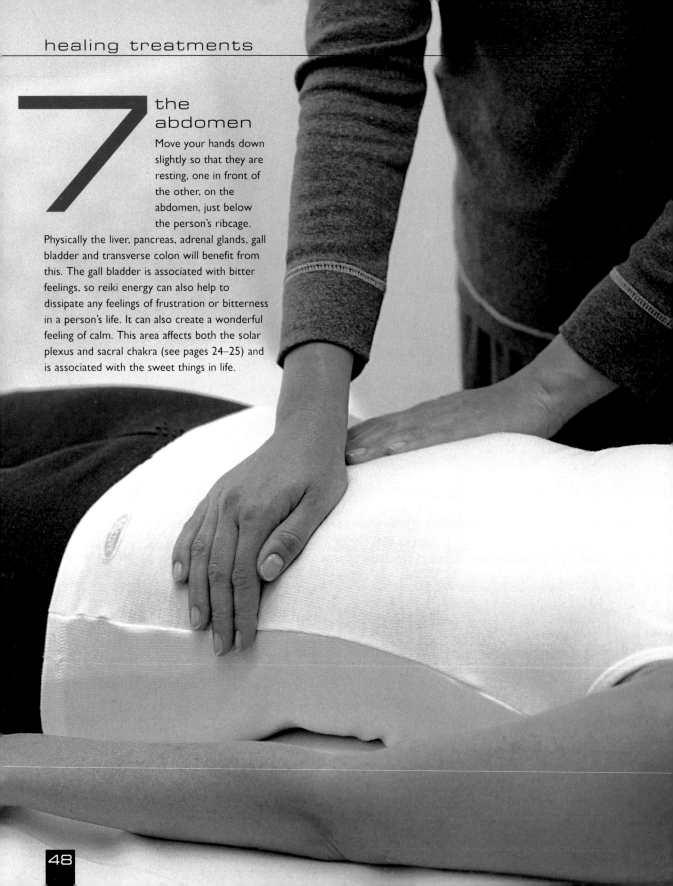

7 the abdomen

Move your hands down slightly so that they are resting, one in front of the other, on the abdomen, just below the person's ribcage. Physically the liver, pancreas, adrenal glands, gall bladder and transverse colon will benefit from this. The gall bladder is associated with bitter feelings, so reiki energy can also help to dissipate any feelings of frustration or bitterness in a person's life. It can also create a wonderful feeling of calm. This area affects both the solar plexus and sacral chakra (see pages 24–25) and is associated with the sweet things in life.

self-treatment

Working on your abdomen
Move your hands down your body slightly so that they rest on either side of your abdomen. Always remember to keep your fingers and thumbs together. The same areas and ailments will be affected as detailed on page 48. Emotionally, the energy can release any stored negativity and help you to realize that you do have control of your life. Often you create experiences in order to learn from them, and by clearing this area, you open yourself up to receive joy and happiness in your life. The reiki energy also helps to bring about balance, physically, mentally and emotionally, as well as creating harmony everywhere in your body.

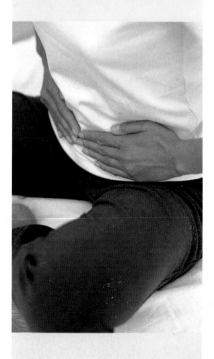

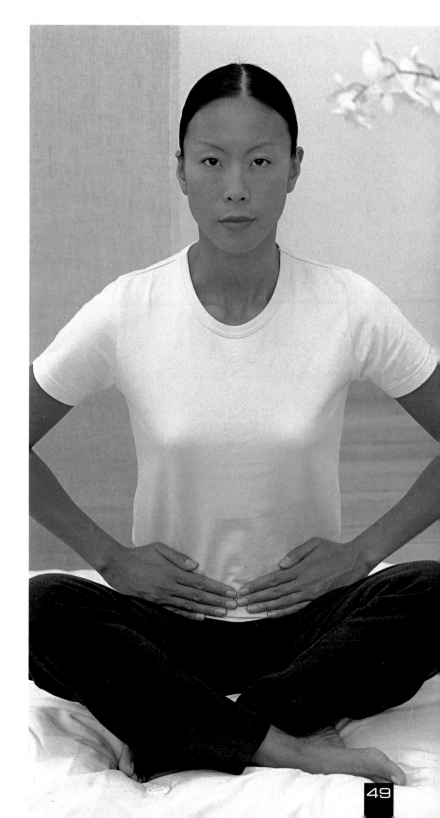

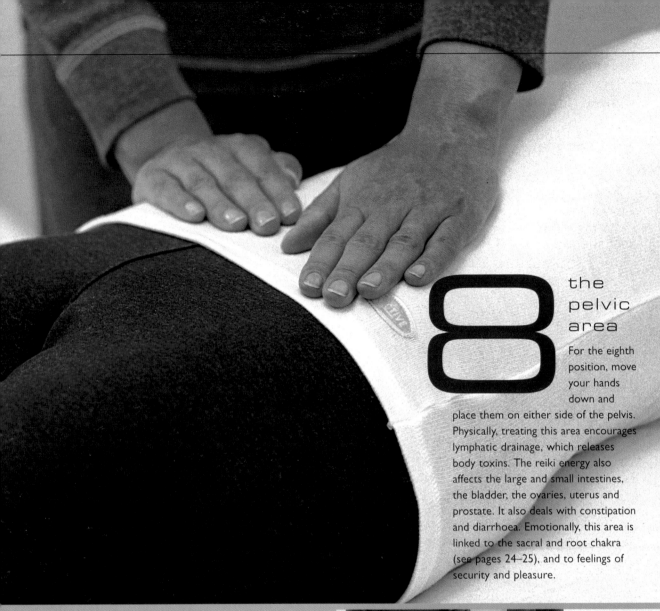

8 the pelvic area

For the eighth position, move your hands down and place them on either side of the pelvis. Physically, treating this area encourages lymphatic drainage, which releases body toxins. The reiki energy also affects the large and small intestines, the bladder, the ovaries, uterus and prostate. It also deals with constipation and diarrhoea. Emotionally, this area is linked to the sacral and root chakra (see pages 24–25), and to feelings of security and pleasure.

treating the knees

Although not officially a traditional position, it is helpful to treat a person's knees by placing one hand on each knee for a few minutes. This area can hold a lot of anger and old emotions, so giving energy here can be very soothing. If you sense that extra time is needed, just hold the position for a bit longer.

treating the feet

Move the energy down from the knees to the feet and hold both ankles for a few minutes, working towards the toes. This helps to move the energy to the bottom of the person's body before you ask them to turn over, so that you can treat their back and shoulders.

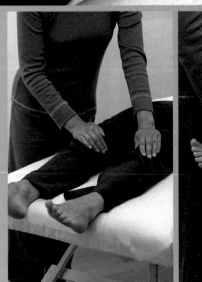
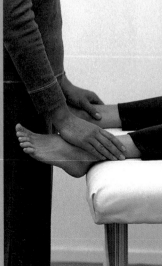

self-treatment

Working on your pelvic area
For this final position on your front, move your hands to your pelvic region and place them on either side of your groin. The same areas and conditions will be affected or helped as mentioned on page 50. Mentally this is also the creative area, where you let go of outmoded ideas or substances that no longer serve any purpose and replace them with feelings that can help you to express yourself. It is here that sexual pleasure, or frustration and guilt is shown. Resentment of a partner also stems from here. You don't need to treat your knees separately as described on the opposite page because when you treat yourself, the reiki energy flows swiftly down your body, but if you have knee problems, you can treat them for a few minutes.

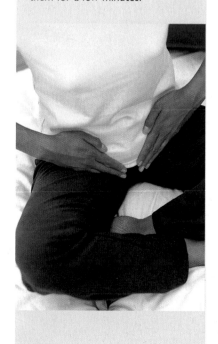

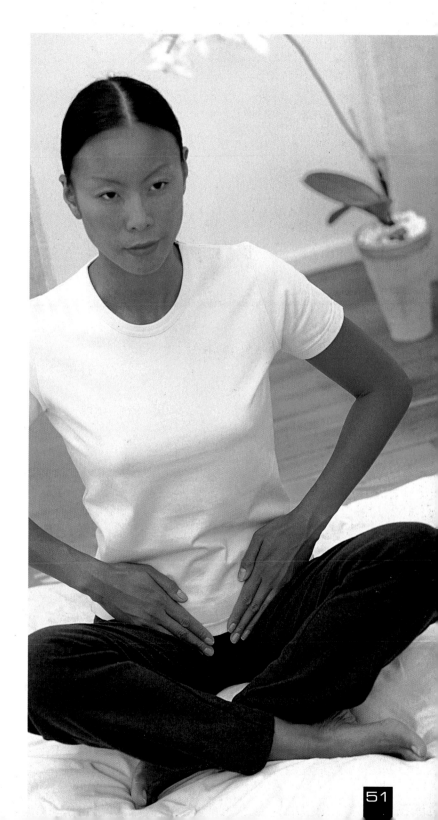

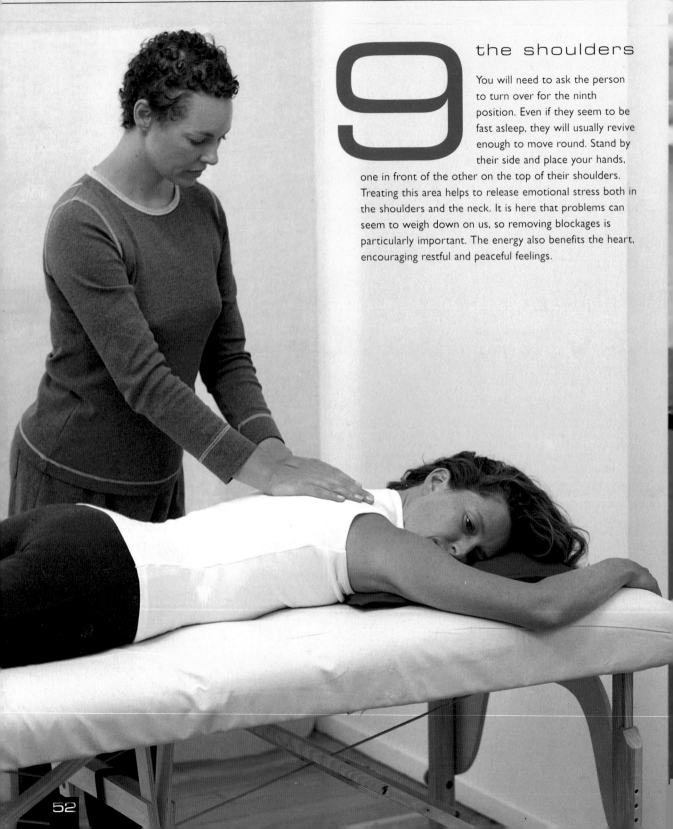

9 the shoulders

You will need to ask the person to turn over for the ninth position. Even if they seem to be fast asleep, they will usually revive enough to move round. Stand by their side and place your hands, one in front of the other on the top of their shoulders. Treating this area helps to release emotional stress both in the shoulders and the neck. It is here that problems can seem to weigh down on us, so removing blockages is particularly important. The energy also benefits the heart, encouraging restful and peaceful feelings.

self-treatment

Working on your shoulders

This is the position where you begin work on the back of your body. Without taking your hands off your body, put your arms behind you and your hands on the top of your shoulders, on either side of your head (shown right). The same areas and ailments will be affected or helped as mentioned on page 52. When you are feeling stressed, try placing your hands on your shoulders, take long, slow deep breaths, and remind yourself to relax. You should feel tension dissipating as the energy flows to this area. This is also helpful when taking a break from a concentrated session at a computer or after being hunched in one position for a while.

Working on your neck and shoulders

You can also try this alternative position (below) which treats the same areas and ailments as mentioned above. Instead of placing your hands on your shoulders, put them on either side of your neck. This also helps to relieve tension at the top of your spinal column and shoulders.

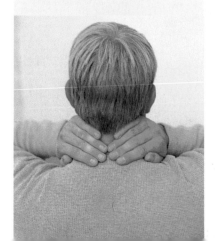

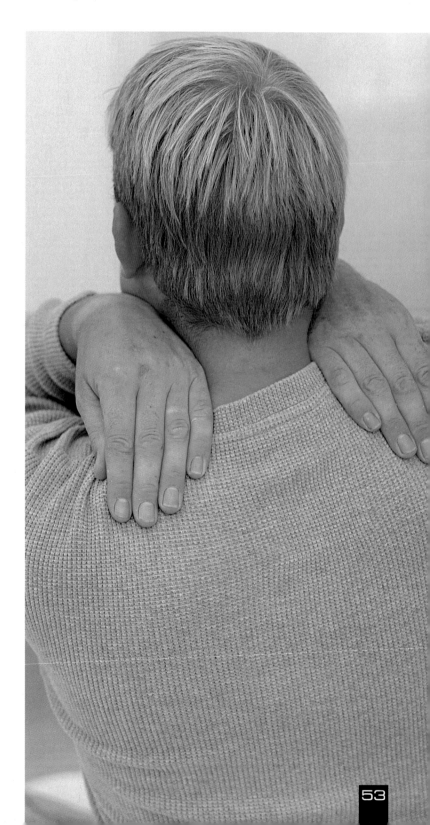

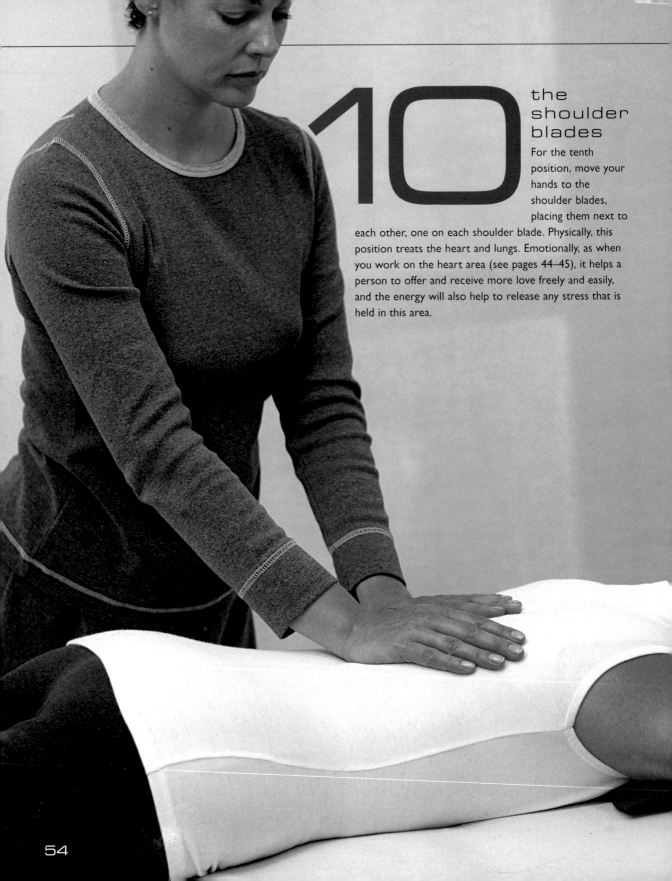

10 the shoulder blades

For the tenth position, move your hands to the shoulder blades, placing them next to each other, one on each shoulder blade. Physically, this position treats the heart and lungs. Emotionally, as when you work on the heart area (see pages 44–45), it helps a person to offer and receive more love freely and easily, and the energy will also help to release any stress that is held in this area.

self-treatment

Working on your shoulder blades (from the back)

To treat your shoulder blades, you need to work on this area in two stages. First put your left hand on your right shoulder, while taking your right hand, palm up, behind you so that it touches your middle back (shown right) and hold for 2½ minutes. To intensify the energy, you can turn the palm on your back to face inwards, but this requires some agility. Then reverse this position, placing your right hand on your left shoulder and your left hand on your middle back, palm up, (shown far right) and hold for 2½ minutes. The same areas and ailments will be affected or helped as detailed on page 54.

Working on your shoulder area (from the front)

If you have an injury or just find it difficult to reach around to your back, you can do this position from the front without affecting the flow of energy. First put your left hand on your right shoulder, place your right hand around your waist (shown right) and hold for 2½ minutes. Then do the position in reverse, putting your right hand on your left shoulder, while placing your left hand around your waist (shown far right) and hold for 2½ minutes.

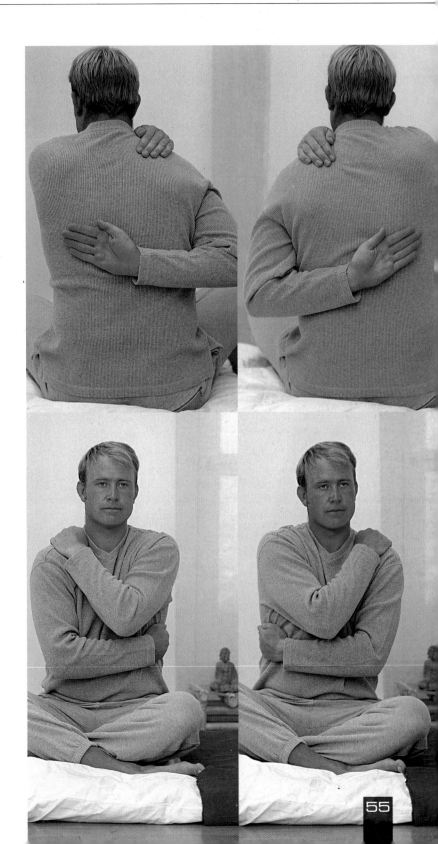

11

the lower back

For the eleventh position, move your hands down to the lower back, placing them one in front of the other near the person's waistband. When the energy flows into this area, its physical effects will cover the gall bladder, pancreas, transverse colon, the adrenal glands, the kidneys and the lower back area. Emotionally, it can alleviate self-criticism and anxiety to make way for happier, more positive feelings.

self-treatment

Working on your lower back
Without taking your hands off your body, move them down to your lower back area, placing them, palms down, on each side of your waist (shown right). The same areas and ailments will be affected or helped as detailed on page 56. The lower back can also hold strong negative emotions, and when these are released, life in general becomes brighter, more peaceful and more positive.

Working on your lower back area
An alternative position to treat your lower back is to place your hands on your lower back, one on top of the other which intensifies the flow of energy (shown below). The same areas and conditions will be affected or helped as mentioned above. Pain in the back area is often like a warning bell, alerting you that something is wrong. This pain is often a physical manifestation of suppressed or repressed emotions or thoughts creating resistance in your body, so always try to work out what these emotions are.

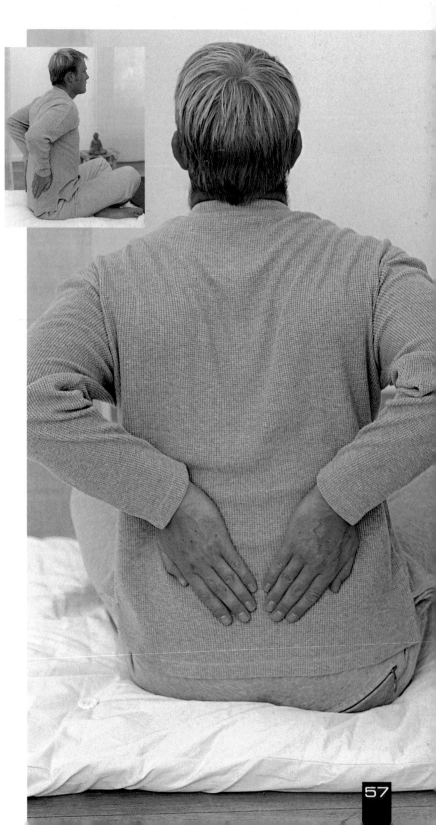

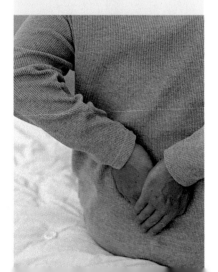

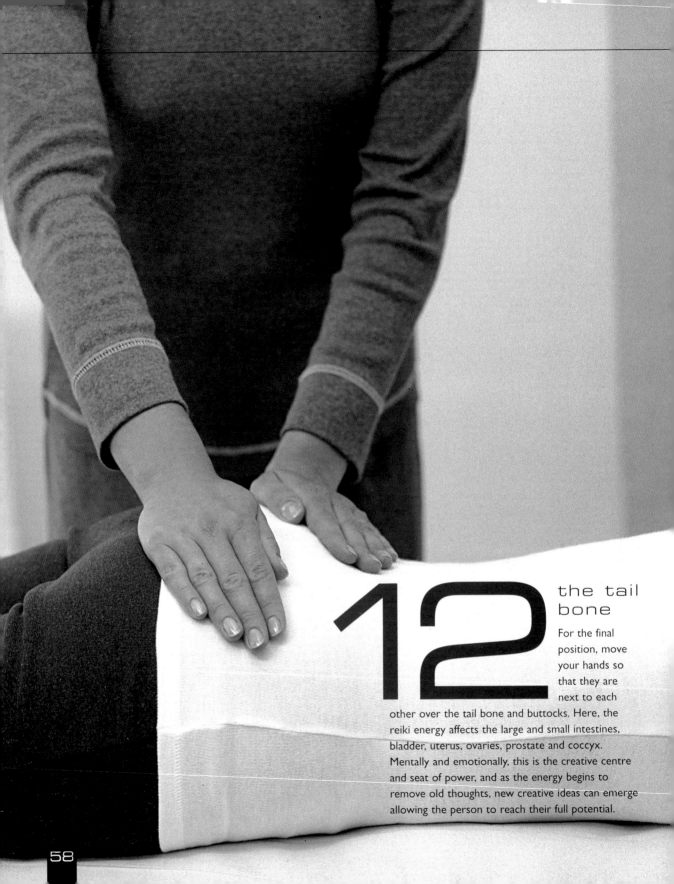

12

the tail bone

For the final position, move your hands so that they are next to each other over the tail bone and buttocks. Here, the reiki energy affects the large and small intestines, bladder, uterus, ovaries, prostate and coccyx. Mentally and emotionally, this is the creative centre and seat of power, and as the energy begins to remove old thoughts, new creative ideas can emerge allowing the person to reach their full potential.

self-treatment

Working on your tail bone

For this last position (shown right) move your hands to either side of your tail bone on your buttocks, so that you are almost sitting on your hands, which should be as close together as possible, or even one on top of the other. The same areas and ailments will be affected or helped as discussed on page 58. Remember that once you have connected to the reiki energy, it will travel to wherever it is needed, encouraging loving, nurturing emotions and helping you to evolve in a positive direction.

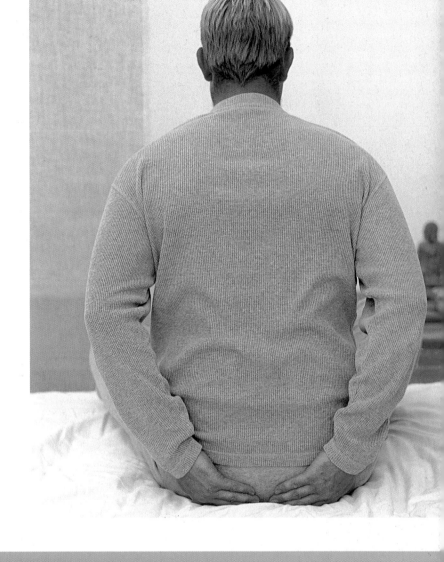

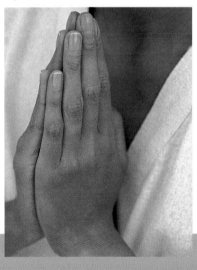

Healing hands – what are you feeling?

During a reiki treatment, your hands may experience a sensation, such as heat or tingling. These feelings can indicate a problem or an area where extra energy is needed. This is a brief guide to interpreting these sensations:

Heat A sign that the energy is particularly needed in this area – heat can often indicate a physical problem.

Coolness There may be an emotional or spiritual blockage indicating the chakra may not be working well.

Tingling This can indicate inflammation in a specific area. If you do not suspect a physical pain, tingling can also point to repressed anger.

Dull pain This normally occurs at the site of an old physical injury or area of scar tissue which might need further healing.

Sharp pain This relates to an area where too much energy is concentrated, causing an imbalance. Working on this area will release the energy.

finishing the treatment

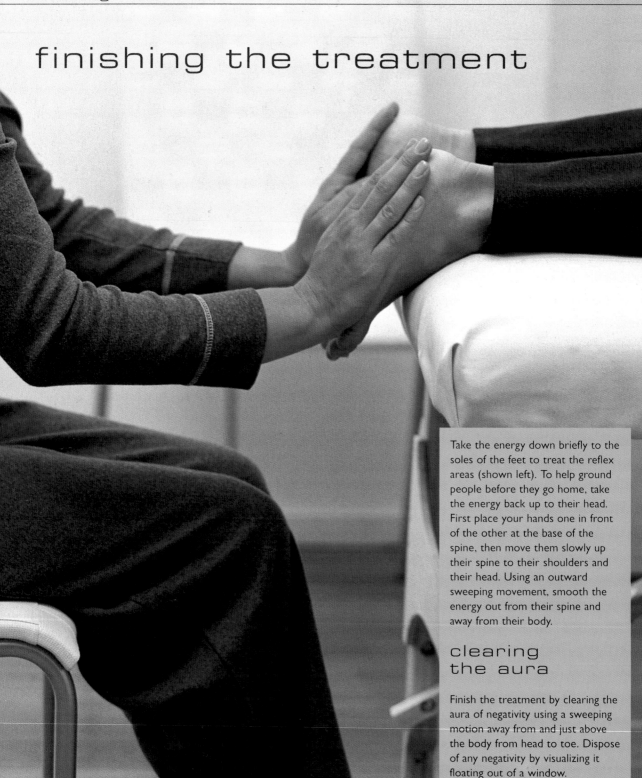

Take the energy down briefly to the soles of the feet to treat the reflex areas (shown left). To help ground people before they go home, take the energy back up to their head. First place your hands one in front of the other at the base of the spine, then move them slowly up their spine to their shoulders and their head. Using an outward sweeping movement, smooth the energy out from their spine and away from their body.

clearing the aura

Finish the treatment by clearing the aura of negativity using a sweeping motion away from and just above the body from head to toe. Dispose of any negativity by visualizing it floating out of a window.

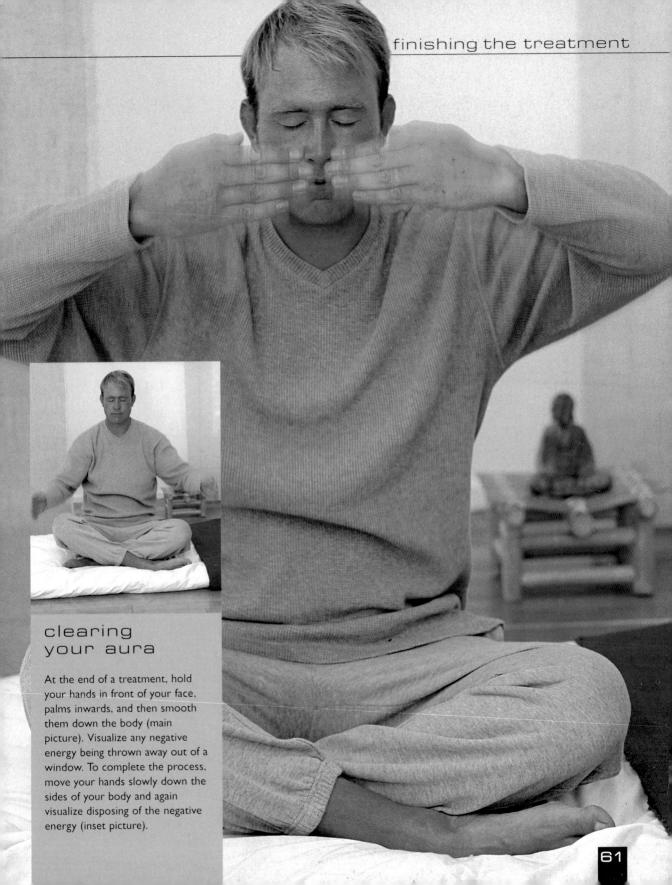

clearing your aura

At the end of a treatment, hold your hands in front of your face, palms inwards, and then smooth them down the body (main picture). Visualize any negative energy being thrown away out of a window. To complete the process, move your hands slowly down the sides of your body and again visualize disposing of the negative energy (inset picture).

Reiki energy is ideal to use to relieve your own or some one else's pain or discomfort when

they are suffering from common or minor ailments. It also combines well with medical or

other complementary treatments.

soothing headaches and migraines

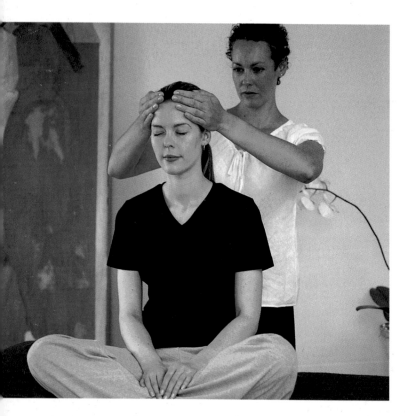

We all suffer from occasional or recurrent headaches or migraines, which can at the least be irritating, or at worst, debilitating. They are often caused by tension, bad posture, hangovers, allergies, eyestrain and neck and spine problems, but reiki healing applied to the painful areas can give soothing relief. Chronic headaches should, however, always be investigated by a doctor.

Treating pain at the top of the head
To treat a headache, ask the person to sit or lie down on a comfortable surface (see pages 30–33). Standing behind them, tune into the energy as you would for the first head position (see page 36) and place the palms of your hands on the side of their head to cover their temples as shown above. Hold for 10–15 minutes or longer until they feel

some relief from the pain. Migraines will normally need several full-body treatments to treat the condition fully and you should try to begin with 3–4 treatments a week, but for some immediate relief from an attack, use the position shown here, treating the ears for a short time (see page 65) and also the solar plexus area (see pages 46–47) to help the person relax and re-balance.

Treating the neck

If the headache stems from the neck or seems to emanate from a specific part of the head, treat this area for a short time as well, putting one hand on top of the other to intensify the flow of energy, as shown below.

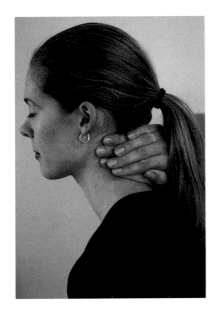

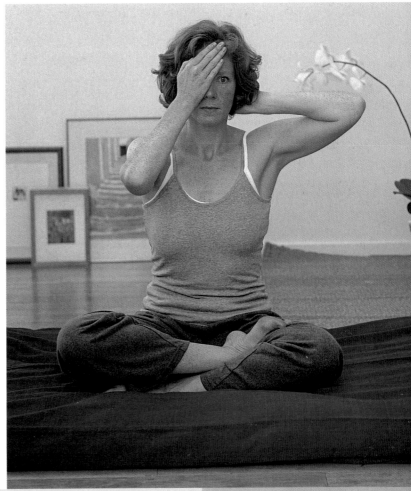

self-treatment

Treating your head

To treat a painful headache, sit on a comfortable surface or a chair. Tune into the energy in the first head position (see page 36) and try to relax by breathing in and out deeply. Place your right hand on your forehead and your left hand on the back of your neck (shown top right), where a lot of muscular tension accumulates. Hold for about 10 minutes, or as long as is comfortable, until you feel the pain lifting.

Treating a specific area

You can also treat a specific area of pain as mentioned above, by putting one hand on top of the other to intensify the healing energy. Here the right temple is receiving the benefit of the healing energy (shown right). Migraines will need more treatment as described on page 62, but use this position to alleviate an attack, treating also your ears (see page 65) and solar plexus (see pages 46–47).

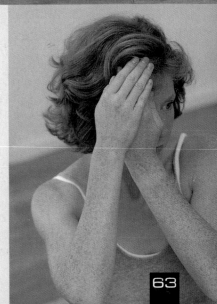

relieving toothache and earache

Bad earache or toothache are often two of the most unpleasant minor ailments that we can experience. The pain from either can be excruciating and treatment from a doctor or dentist should be sought quickly, but a reiki session can bring fast relief from suffering.

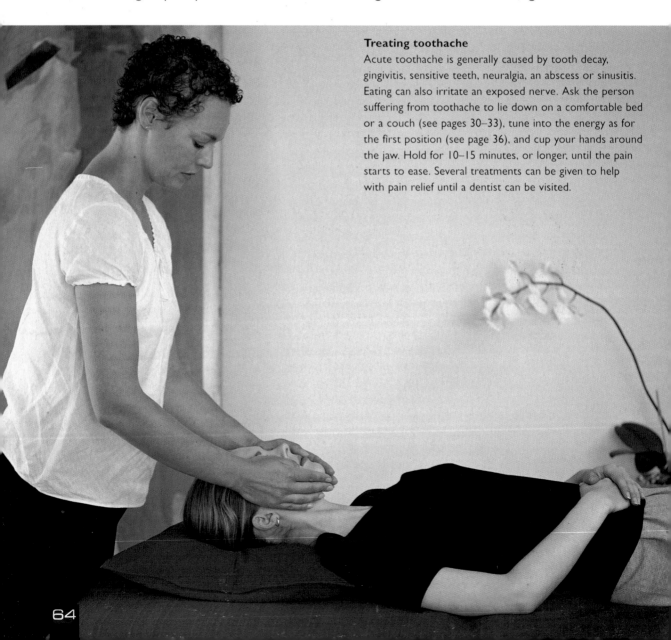

Treating toothache
Acute toothache is generally caused by tooth decay, gingivitis, sensitive teeth, neuralgia, an abscess or sinusitis. Eating can also irritate an exposed nerve. Ask the person suffering from toothache to lie down on a comfortable bed or a couch (see pages 30–33), tune into the energy as for the first position (see page 36), and cup your hands around the jaw. Hold for 10–15 minutes, or longer, until the pain starts to ease. Several treatments can be given to help with pain relief until a dentist can be visited.

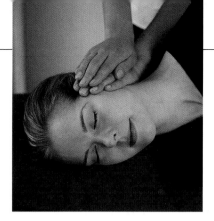

Treating earache

The outer, middle and inner ear can all become inflamed or infected with either bacteria or a virus. Swimming in polluted water or having a bad cold or flu can cause infection for both adults and children. To treat someone with bad earache, ask them to lie on their side on a bed or comfortable sofa with the affected side facing up. Tune into the energy as for the first head position (see page 36), and place your hands, palms down, one on top of the other on the affected ear drum for 10–15 minutes, or until the pain is alleviated.

self-treatment

Easing earache

To relieve a painful ear infection, sit on a comfortable surface or a chair. Tune into the healing energy as in the first head position (see page 36) and place your hands, one on top of the other on the infected ear (shown right). Hold for 10–15 minutes, or until you can feel the pain subsiding.

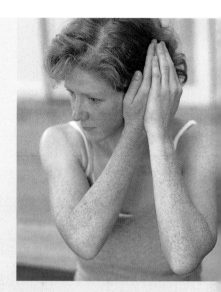

Relieving toothache

To alleviate the pain from an inflamed tooth or teeth, lie down on a padded surface, resting your jaw on your hands, keeping them placed one on top of the other to increase the intensity of the energy (shown below). Hold this position for 10–15 minutes, or for as long as you need. Your hands may become warm or even hot – reiki energy can feel very hot when you are treating an injury – this is a sign that the energy is being drawn into the inflamed area. Keep working on the area until you feel the ache begin to ebb away. Continue treatment every couple of days until you can visit a dentist.

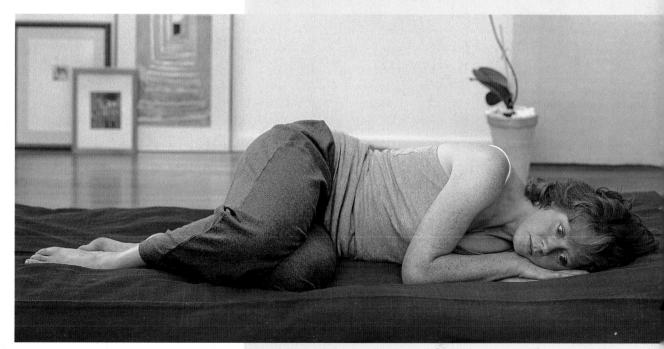

easing back pain

Most back pain is muscular and the following sequence of treatments can ease the discomfort, but should not be attempted if there is a spinal injury, or if you suspect one. Many negative thoughts about ourselves are stored in the back and reiki healing energy can gently release these beliefs and relieve the pain.

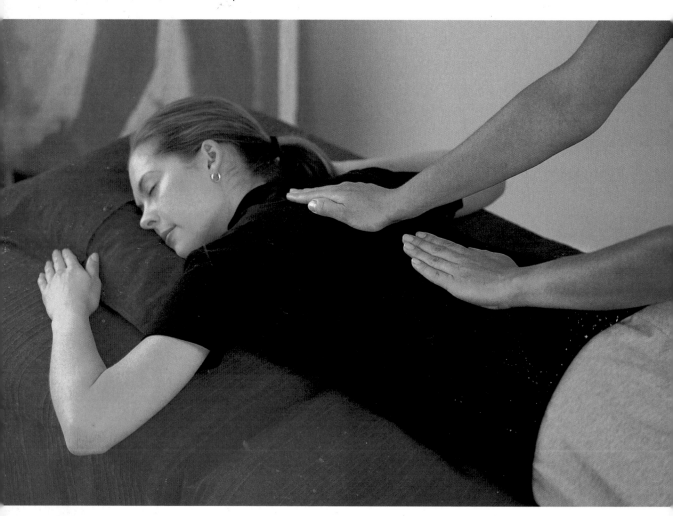

1 Ask the person to lie flat on their stomach on a comfortable, padded surface or massage table. Tune into the energy as you would for the first head position (see page 36), then place your hands at the top of their spine with one hand positioned above the other.

Hold this position for a couple of minutes and then move one hand down at a time to the bottom of the spine, holding each position for a couple of minutes. This will relax their spine, allowing it to come into alignment, and, in the process, free the flow of healing energy.

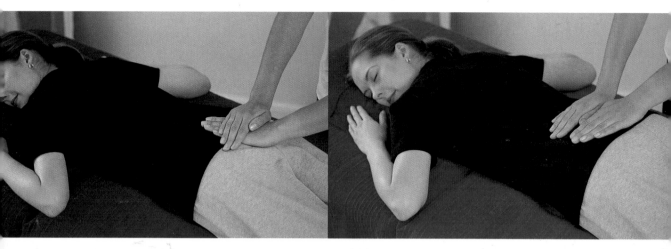

2 Place your hands on top of each other at the bottom of their spine as shown, and hold for a couple of minutes, allowing the energy at the base of their spine to move upwards. This position will help to release any long-held muscular tension and provide some "grounding" energy to balance the effects of any release of strong emotions stored in the area.

These treatments are only recommended for people with minor back problems. If serious back pain is experienced a doctor, osteopath or chiropractor should always be consulted first.

3 Place your hands on the sacrum (the large flat bone in the lower back) as shown and hold for a couple of minutes to let the healing energy flow. This position is very good for lower back pain, problems with the sciatic nerve and leg pain. To finish and balance the energy in the back, put your right hand between the person's shoulder blades and then your left hand on their lower back, keeping contact with the person's body with one hand while moving the other. This will help keep the reiki energy flowing smoothly and uninterrupted. Hold this position briefly to calm the muscles and increase the spinal energy flow.

self-treatment

Treating your back

Lie down on a comfortable surface with your knees raised slightly. Place your left hand on your midriff with your right hand just below it on your pelvis. Breathe in and out slowly and deeply, allowing yourself to "connect" with your back for at least 5 minutes. The floor will support your back and as the reiki takes effect minor realignments will occur naturally. This is a very relaxing treatment that is excellent for relieving muscular tension and physical exhaustion. Be prepared for a release of deep emotion as the body cells may let go of unhappy memories that have been stored there. Reiki always operates for your highest good, so it will not encourage emotional release that needs another person's support.

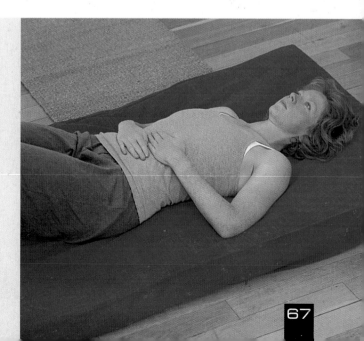

helping breathing problems

Colds, flu and minor chest infections are common during the winter months. They can cause lung congestion and breathing difficulties which can be relieved by reiki treatments. Chronic illnesses such as bronchitis and asthma can also improve with regular reiki sessions.

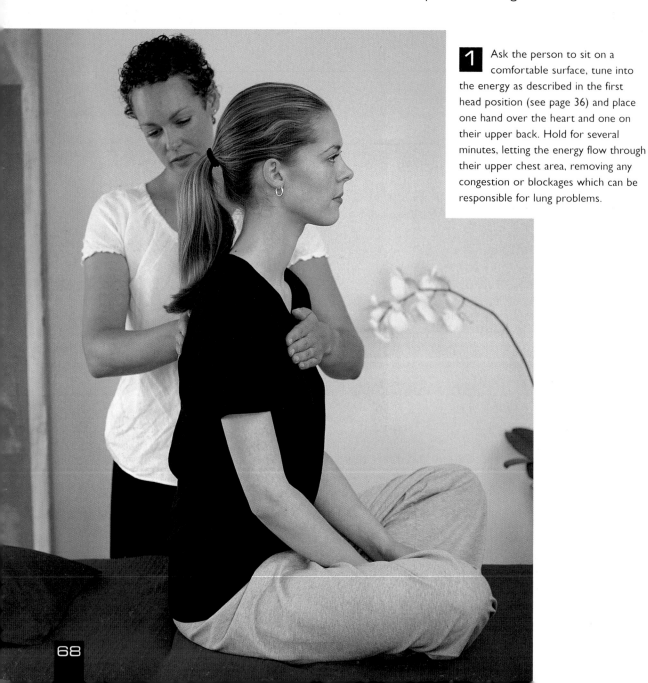

1 Ask the person to sit on a comfortable surface, tune into the energy as described in the first head position (see page 36) and place one hand over the heart and one on their upper back. Hold for several minutes, letting the energy flow through their upper chest area, removing any congestion or blockages which can be responsible for lung problems.

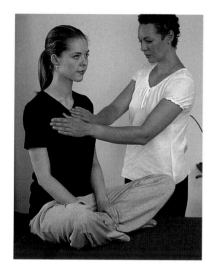

2 Place your hands side by side on at the top of their chest area and hold for a few minutes. Then move down a hand width and repeat. Feel the energy moving through their lungs and balancing them by clearing blockages and freeing the airways. The person's breathing may now also start to increase or slow down slightly – a sign that the energy is taking effect. Carry on in this way until you have treated the whole chest area.

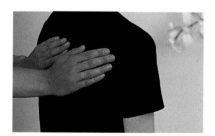

3 Now work on the back, placing your hands on their upper back. Hold for a few minutes, then move down their back a hand width at a time as above until you have covered all the lung area. You can also treat the sides in the same way to energize the whole lung system; this is easier to do if the person is lying down on their side.

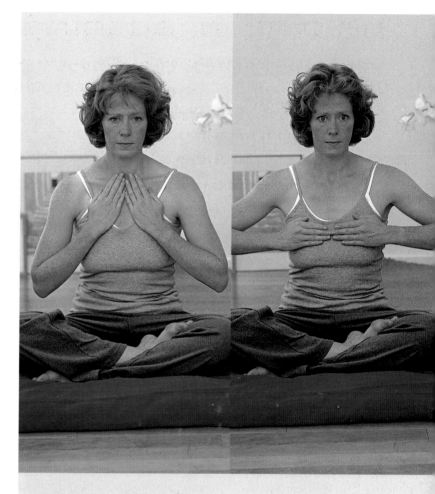

self-treatment

1 To treat yourself, sit comfortably on a padded surface. Tune into the energy as described in the first head position (see page 36) and try to relax. Either place your hands, palms down either side of your heart area or pointing upwards towards your throat (as shown top left), which can be more comfortable. Hold for several minutes, letting the energy work through your blocked lungs and chest.

2 Now move your hands a hand width down your chest, placing them on either side (shown top right). Again hold for a few minutes, or until you feel the strength of the energy dissipating. Carry on in the same way until you have covered the entire chest area and start to feel some easing of pressure. Working on your own back can prove awkward, but for extra benefit you can place your hands on the sides of your body and work down the same area.

69

boosting the immune system and circulation

Periods of prolonged stress can affect the immune system making people tired and vulnerable to viral infections as well as more serious illnesses. Poor blood circulation can restrict the efficiency of the lymphatic system causing sluggishness and toxic build-up. Reiki healing applied directly to all these areas can greatly improve their functioning.

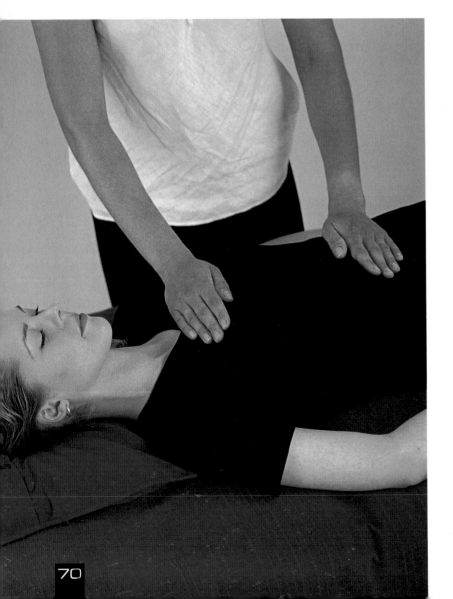

Treating the immune system
Ask the person to lie down on a comfortable padded surface (see pages 30–33). Stand at their side and tune into the energy as described in the first head position (see page 36). Place one hand over the heart on the upper chest and place the other one on the abdomen, slightly to the left over the spleen. Hold this position for 10–15 minutes. Working intensively on the heart area stimulates the immune system, while working on the abdomen boosts the spleen function and helps to fight infection. Repeating this treatment three or four times a week at first will normally prove very beneficial. Once improvement has begun, you can scale down the frequency of treatment.

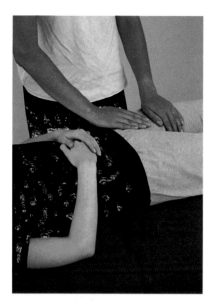

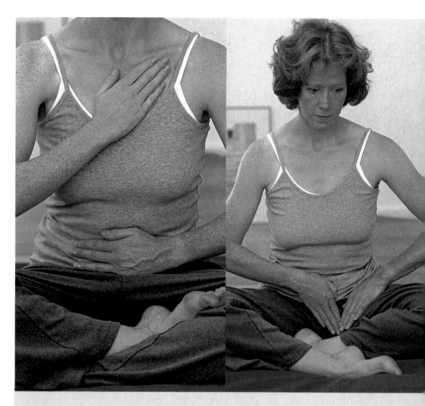

Treating the lymphatic system

To treat poor blood circulation, ask the person to lie down on a comfortable padded surface (see pages 30–33) and work first on their legs. Tune into the energy as described in the first head position on page 36 and place your left hand on the top of their left inner thigh and your right hand on their groin and hold for 10 minutes, allowing the energy to penetrate the arteries. Then change hands, placing your right hand on their right inner thigh and the left hand on their groin and again hold this position for 10 minutes. You can also treat the lymph glands in the armpits by placing your hands side by side around each armpit. Again hold for 10 minutes, then treat the other armpit. This will really aid toxic release, so warn the person you are treating about this as their body will suddenly become more effective in releasing waste material and detoxifying itself.

self-treatment

Treating your immune system

To treat yourself, sit comfortably on a padded surface and tune into the energy as described in the first head position (see page 36). Place your right hand, pointing upwards over your chest and heart area and place your left hand on your abdomen – keep it slightly to the left to cover the spleen (shown top left). Hold this position for about 10–15 minutes, letting the energy work through your immune system and spleen, as described on the opposite page, to help them to operate more efficiently.

Treating your lymphatic system

If you have poor blood circulation or problems with your lymphatic system, sit comfortably on a padded surface and tune into the energy as described on page 36. Place your left hand on your inner left thigh and your right hand on your groin (shown top right) and hold for 10 minutes, feeling the energy stimulating the blood circulation in this area. Then place your right hand on your right inner thigh and your left on the groin and again hold for 10 minutes. You can also treat your lymph glands in your armpits by placing your hands on top of each other in these areas. Hold each side for about 10 minutes. Be prepared for a physical clear out of toxins as the body will start to eliminate any accumulated waste.

alleviating stress

Stress is a modern problem that affects everybody, both at work and at home. Some stress is essential for stimulation, but when it overwhelms our coping mechanisms, it can seriously affect our health. Reiki can help to calm the nervous system and soothe the adrenal glands, which provokes our "fight or flight" reaction to stress.

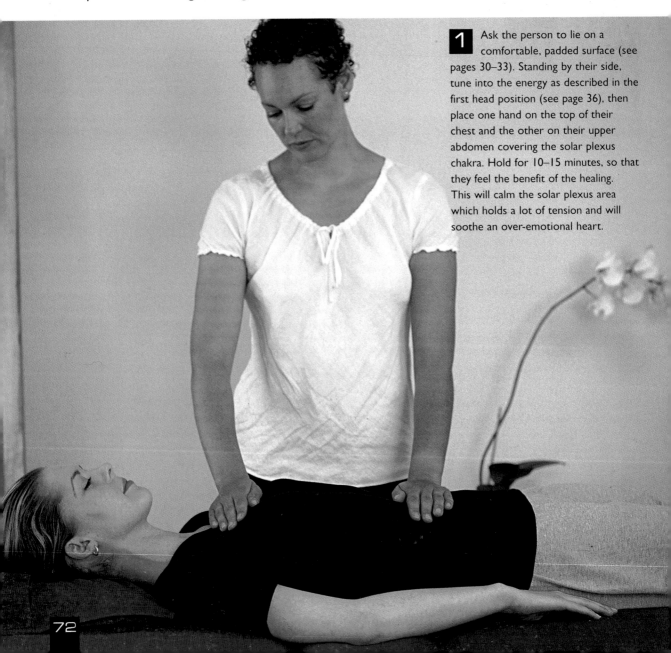

1 Ask the person to lie on a comfortable, padded surface (see pages 30–33). Standing by their side, tune into the energy as described in the first head position (see page 36), then place one hand on the top of their chest and the other on their upper abdomen covering the solar plexus chakra. Hold for 10–15 minutes, so that they feel the benefit of the healing. This will calm the solar plexus area which holds a lot of tension and will soothe an over-emotional heart.

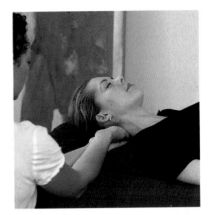

2 With the person still lying down, move around to their other side and sitting down, put your hands one on top of the other under the back of their head. Hold for 10–15 minutes, or for as long as you feel is needed. This is similar to the nurturing position on page 40 and will release the tension held here. It will also reduce stress levels and induce a feeling of relaxation.

self-treatment

1 If you are feeling stressed or tense, sit on a comfortable, padded surface or a chair. Tune into the energy as in the first head position (see page 36) and calm yourself by breathing in and out deeply for a few minutes. Place one hand on your chest over your heart and put the other one on your upper abdomen over the solar plexus chakra (shown top right). Hold this position for 10–15 minutes, feeling the release of any tension. You will find that you will become energized and revitalized and will become more resilient and able to cope with life.

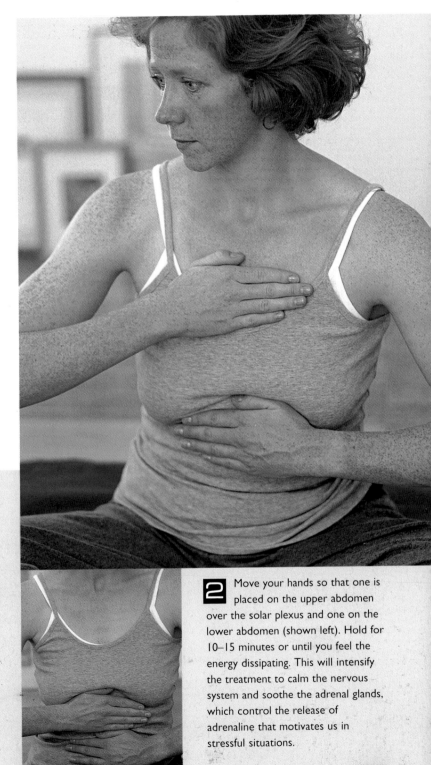

2 Move your hands so that one is placed on the upper abdomen over the solar plexus and one on the lower abdomen (shown left). Hold for 10–15 minutes or until you feel the energy dissipating. This will intensify the treatment to calm the nervous system and soothe the adrenal glands, which control the release of adrenaline that motivates us in stressful situations.

73

case histories

NAME: Eleanor

REASON FOR
TREATMENT:
depression, had
lost the zest
for life

NUMBER OF REIKI
SESSIONS:
12

Eleanor had reached the age of 40 and felt very depressed about the future when she first sought reiki treatment after a recommendation from a friend. She had a series of 12 treatments which she felt helped to re-focus her life. During each treatment, Eleanor could feel heat and a tingling sensation coming from the healer's hands, and she also came to believe that she was loved unconditionally. At the end of each treatment she felt light-headed and very thirsty, which is quite a common experience. Physically, she experienced extreme nausea when her abdomen was treated, which disappeared when the healer removed her hands – this was the area where she was suffering from fibroids and the nausea was an indicator of emotions that needed to be released.

Emotionally, Eleanor also felt a tremendous release of emotions and cried during many of the sessions. She felt the need to forgive and to be forgiven and began to sleep deeply, experiencing vivid dreams about her past life. There seemed to be "homework" to do after each session and Eleanor spent a lot of time thinking about herself and her relationships with other people.

Eleanor is convinced that reiki has helped her to find her true self. She feels that it has helped her marriage as well as how she deals with other people. Eleanor has now gone on to take Reiki I and II herself and now treats other people.

W hen Kenneth first went for a reiki treatment, he was still recovering from M.E. after suffering from it for six very difficult years. At each healing session, he was very aware of the healer's hands as they moved through the body positions and also felt some heat or tingling sensations. He also experienced a strange floating feeling. Physically he felt his body functions were slowing down, but mentally he became much more clear-headed. Emotionally he felt a greater awareness of himself, experiencing feelings of gratitude and relief that he was finally moving forward both physically and mentally. The reiki treatments enabled him to come to terms with his illness and the limitations it imposed on him.

Kenneth felt immediate physical and emotional benefits after his first reiki treatment, which progressively increased with subsequent sessions. He feels he is on the road to recovery now and is still receiving reiki treatments accompanied by aromatherapy massage. He also feels for the first time that there is a positive end in sight for him.

NAME: Kenneth

REASON FOR TREATMENT: recovering from M.E. (myalgic encephalomyelitis or chronic fatigue syndrome)

NUMBER OF REIKI SESSIONS: numerous

NAME: James

REASON FOR
TREATMENT:
extreme pain
from spinal
problems

NUMBER OF REIKI
SESSIONS:
minimum of
6 treatments

James was in his mid-60s when he underwent an operation on his spine to resolve long-term back problems, but the operation was not a success and he ended up being confined to a wheelchair for two years. He then tried some Bowen technique sessions (a form of body work) which helped him to walk again, albeit painfully. When he had his first reiki treatment he felt a very strong tingling sensation at the base of spine. This was particularly strong when the healer worked on his shoulders as the energy was travelling right down his spinal cord.

Physically, after his first treatment, James's pain lessened for the first time in six years. Naturally, he felt elated and very emotional that the healing could have had such a powerful effect so quickly.

James then went for several more reiki sessions and the positive effect of the energy was accumulative. He soon found that he was able to climb stairs again – something that he had not done in years. He feels reiki has improved his spinal condition considerably and enabled him to walk properly again.

Lenny in his mid-70s, had suffered regularly from both migraines and asthma all his life. He decided to try reiki because some of his family had enjoyed successful reiki treatments. Although sceptical at first, he soon relaxed into the treatments, normally falling asleep during the sessions. He often felt a strong heat through the healer's hands and a tingling sensation in his toes as the energy worked its way right through his body. After a few treatments, he realized he was no longer suffering from migraines and that he didn't need to use his asthma inhaler any more. Lenny also became much more tolerant and less judgemental of people. He is now a warmer, more open person, able to express his feelings and emotions freely.

NAME: Lenny

REASON FOR TREATMENT: migraines and asthma

NUMBER OF REIKI SESSIONS: 6

John had suffered from high blood pressure for many years and took strong medication to keep it under control. He decided to try reiki to help his condition, and felt a lot of heat from the healer's hands when he was being worked on as well as becoming more relaxed than he had been for ages. After only a couple of reiki treatments, he had to visit his specialist for a check-up, and the specialist was amazed to find that for the first time in years John's blood pressure was beginning to come down. The improvement continued after several more healing sessions and in fact, John has now managed to come off medication completely. He has also gone on to take Reiki I and II so that he can treat himself regularly.

NAME: John

REASON FOR TREATMENT: high blood pressure

NUMBER OF REIKI SESSIONS: on-going treatments to control his blood pressure

reiki for babies and children

Reiki is a wonderful way to strengthen the bond with a new baby and intensify the relationship with the mother and father. It can also help to reduce any trauma associated with a long or painful birth. The healing energy will soothe babies if they are crying, and reduce the uncomfortable symptoms of colic or the inflammation of teething. You can treat them while you are cradling them after a feed, or while they are sleeping. Only a few of the main positions (see pages 36–59), or adaptations, will be necessary as they are so small, and you need only to spend about 5 minutes on the treatment. Simply making contact with their bodies by holding them will pass on the healing energy.

Pregnant women can also gain huge benefit from reiki as it relieves the unpleasant symptoms of morning sickness and also helps to ease lower back pain. The growing baby also seems to enjoy the energy and will often respond with a kick as the reiki treatment is being given. A daily or weekly treatment that concentrates on the abdomen, the heart, the solar plexus and the temples will help the mother-to-be to adjust to all the physical changes that are taking place.

treating children

Children usually enjoy reiki and respond quickly to treatment. They soon learn to ask for a healing first aid session on the affected area if they have a stomach ache or headache (see pages 62–63) or if they have cut or bruised themselves when playing. Often you can just sit them on your lap and treat them while reading a story.

As children are so much smaller they do not need to be treated for a full hour – normally 20 to 30 minutes should be sufficient. They can also get quite hot during treatment, so you should judge how long the session should last, depending on how well the child is receiving the energy. Most children do not yet have the emotional complications that we accumulate as adults, so consequently the healing energy flows much more quickly through them.

Reiki can also help when children need to be calmed down and reassured after experiencing a terrifying nightmare. Place one hand on their forehead with the other on their abdomen over their solar plexus (see page 46), hold for about 5 minutes or until they seem more relaxed.

giving reiki to restless babies and toddlers

Trying to get young children and babies to stay still long enough to give them a full, hour-long treatment can often prove difficult as they often start to wriggle about after a few minutes. You can treat them lying down on a padded surface (see pages 30–33), but if they will not lie still, let them sit up while you treat them and let them talk to you if they want. If your child or baby is really restless, it can often be easier to treat them when they are asleep. You won't be able to follow all the main positions exactly, so just sit by the cot or crib and adapt them as best you can, bearing in mind that the reiki energy will go through all bedding and duvets. Often the beneficial effects are immediate and parents have been amazed how minor problems have been resolved, and how happy and relaxed their children appear the next morning after a reiki treatment.

Obviously, reiki will work particularly well when you are treating your own children as they are already relaxed and comfortable with you, but if you are asked to treat other people's children, try to calm them as much as possible as they may be slightly

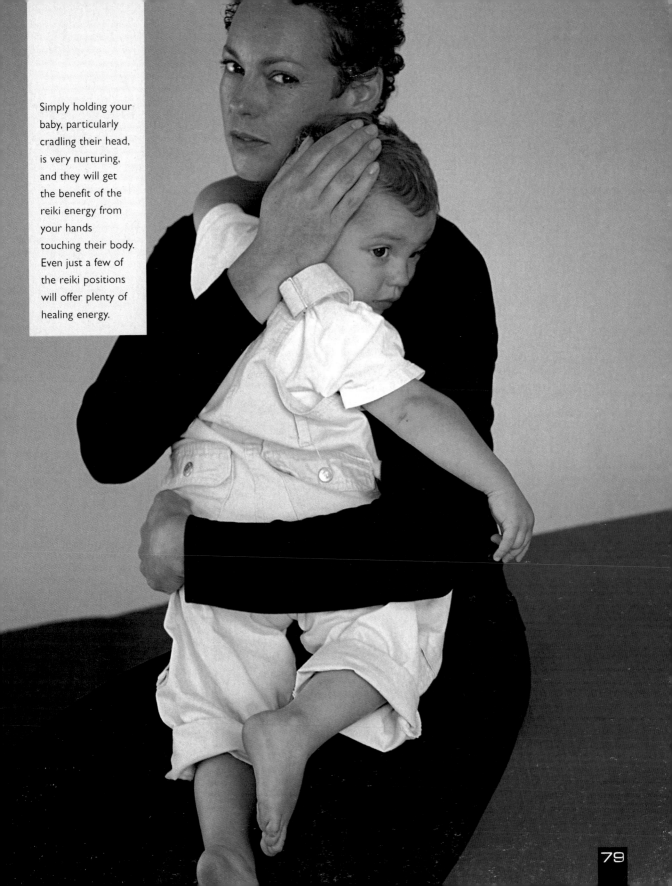

Simply holding your baby, particularly cradling their head, is very nurturing, and they will get the benefit of the reiki energy from your hands touching their body. Even just a few of the reiki positions will offer plenty of healing energy.

apprehensive about what you are going to do. Sometimes you will only be able to use some of the main positions before the child gets bored and wanders off. Older children are normally willing to stay still for a longer time, so you will be able to give them a full-body treatment as for an adult (see pages 36–61) but bear in mind that you will probably need to spend less time in each position. As mentioned before, you will notice how the energy seems to flow faster than adults.

receiving attunements

Children can even receive the reiki attunements from about the age of 8, although you are the best judge of their maturity. So if you are practising reiki, you can get your reiki master to initiate your child. They will also have to go through the 21- or 30-day cleansing period after attunement and you can help them through any emotional or physical upsets. They can then become involved in family treatment sessions, treating you and their other siblings.

beginning a treatment

A good way to relax a child at the start of a reiki session is to put one hand on their heart and the other one behind their head (shown below). This also helps to soothe their mind and emotions.

Older children can be more willing to lie still so that you can work through a full-body treatment over an hour (the seventh position is shown below). Alternatively, you can treat them while they are sleeping.

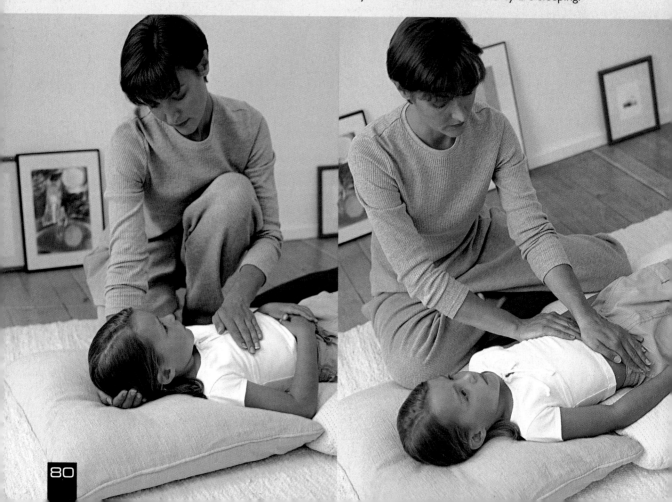

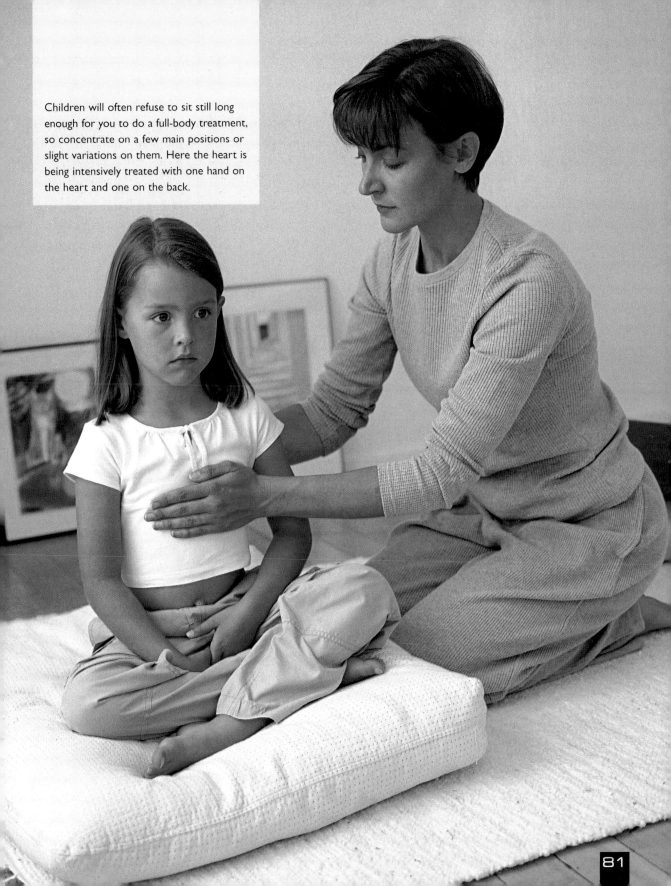

Children will often refuse to sit still long enough for you to do a full-body treatment, so concentrate on a few main positions or slight variations on them. Here the heart is being intensively treated with one hand on the heart and one on the back.

treating the elderly

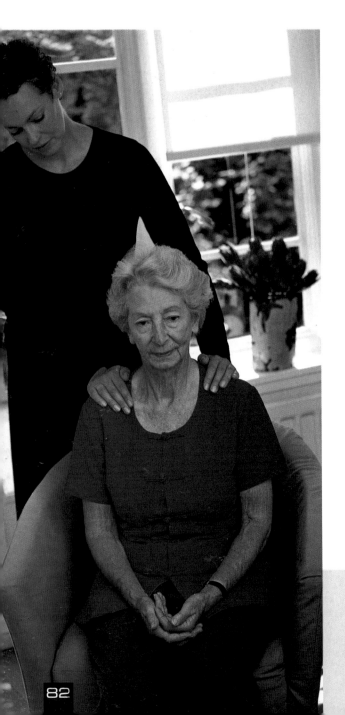

Elderly people may often live on their own, and unless they have a pet, they can often suffer from lack of regular warmth, affection and touch – something that we all need to thrive. The older generation can also be more inhibited and less inclined to go for therapies such as massage or aromatherapy which can involve the removal of some of their clothes. A reiki treatment can be very beneficial as it will help them relax and let them sleep better and longer. It can also ease painful ailments such as arthritis and rheumatism, giving them more mobility and balancing their body functions. A reiki treatment can also be used safely with most medication, and in fact often complements them. Reiki can also be given to the terminally ill and can help them find peace and serenity.

adapting the treatment

Ideally, you should perform the 12 basic positions on an elderly person who is lying down on a comfortable padded surface (see pages 36–61). However, if they are not very mobile and would not be comfortable on the floor or able to climb onto a massage couch, treat them sitting in a chair. You should try to ensure that you can move freely around them so you can treat their sides and back, but if this is not possible, work round as best you can, adapting the hand positions to fit.

Some elderly people find it easier to be treated in a chair, even though it is not as relaxing. Work through the main body positions, paying particular attention to any other areas such as stiff joints that may need attention.

pets and plants

Family pets normally respond very well to reiki and seem to relax almost immediately. They seem to know instinctively how much energy they need and will run off when they feel they have had enough, which may be after just a few minutes. People who treat their pets regularly have even found that they have been able to reduce their vet's bills. As some pets are smaller than humans, it may not be possible to follow the positions exactly.

treating pets

Generally, start where the animal likes to be stroked, placing your hands behind their ears. Cats, however, don't like this position, so try putting one hand on their head and one on their throat. Move onto the other main body areas as you would with humans. Spend longer on any place where the animal seems to experience pain. Sometimes the animal will move during a session, and it may be trying to show you a particular area where it wants treatment.

treating plants

Houseplants respond well to reiki and you can energize the water you give them by putting your hands around the watering can. Alternatively, hold your hands around the base of pot to treat the roots. When you feel enough energy has been absorbed, move your hands up to the leaves and hold them a short distance away for a few minutes. If the plant still does not thrive, move it to another part of the room as it might be suffering from bad positioning.

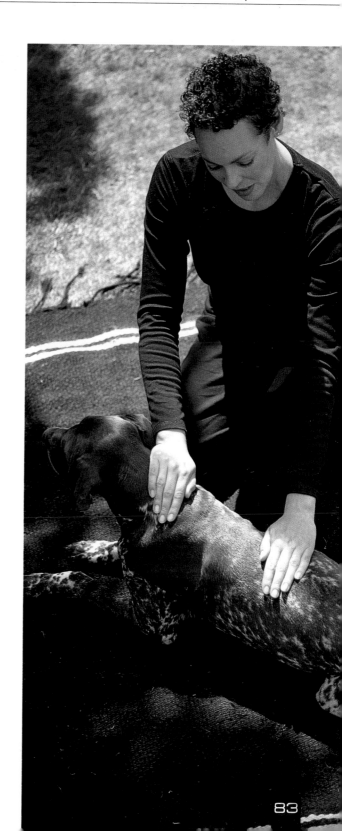

reiki and colour therapy

Reiki works well in combination with other therapies and especially when it is practised with colour therapy to create balance and harmony in the body. Colours are known to have vibratory frequencies which have a profound effect on us and our emotions. Sometimes, we even intuitively wear a colour that we sense our body needs. Illness is believed to be associated with chakras that are imbalanced – not working well – so when reiki is performed with colour therapy, it intensifies the energy sent to the areas that are malfunctioning.

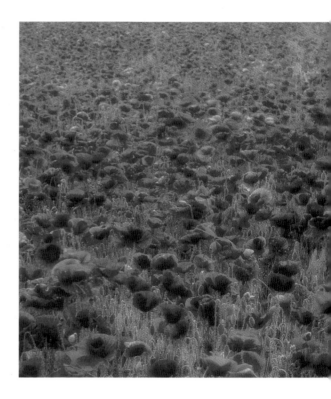

All colours vibrate at different frequencies, so we respond differently to each one. We may also react to a colour because of a previous association – if, for example, you wore a navy blue school uniform, you may well still feel some aversion to that colour. How we react to colour can be linked to our chakras, and obviously, if there are any imbalances in our chakras, there will be emotional reactions as well as physical illness. So if someone is suffering from an underactive thyroid in the throat area, for example, blue (the colour of the throat chakra) is used to harmonize the area. Although there are no firm rules about using colour and combining it with reiki, generally the chakras will respond well to treatment with their relevant colours. You can use any type of material or paper; similarly, the shape or size of the material doesn't matter – it is the colour that is important.

First chakra –
The root (base of spine)
Colour of chakra: red – the colour of passion, strengthens connection to the earth and will to live
Can help: lack of energy or enthusiasm for life

When doing a full-body treatment, place a piece of paper or material that is a soft red colour (bright red can be too energizing) over the root chakra on the pelvic area (see position 8, pages 50–51). Perform the reiki on the paper or material in the usual way for 5 minutes, or for as long as you feel the energy is needed. Channelling reiki through the colour intensifies the energy, helping to equalize the chakra area. If you don't want to use material or paper you can just visualize the colour going to the chakra.

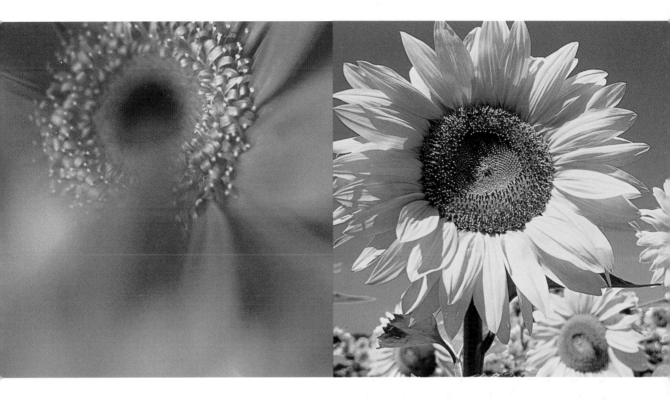

Second chakra –
The sacral (pelvic area)
Colour of chakra: orange – a more gentle colour,
associated with joy and happiness, will increase
sexual energy and boost immune system
Can help: kidney and bladder problems,
poor intuitive abilities, sexual dysfunction

During a full-body treatment, place an orange-
coloured piece of paper or material on the sacral
chakra over the lower abdomen (see position 7,
pages 48–49). Perform the reiki on the paper or
material for 5 minutes or until the energy dissipates.
As mentioned before, you can visualize the colour
going to the chakra as you do the reiki instead of
using a physical symbol of colour.

Third chakra –
The solar plexus (upper abdomen)
Colour of chakra: yellow – a warm, soothing
colour, helps to clear the mind and aid learning,
creates a feeling of what is right and just
Can help: mood swings, depression, poor digestion
and nervous problems

When performing a full-body treatment, place a
yellow piece of paper or material over the solar
plexus on the upper abdomen (see position 6, pages
46–47). Place your hands on the paper or material as
you do the reiki for 5 minutes or for as long as
necessary. Alternatively, if you haven't got anything in
the correct colour, you can visualize the colour
influencing the chakra as you do the reiki.

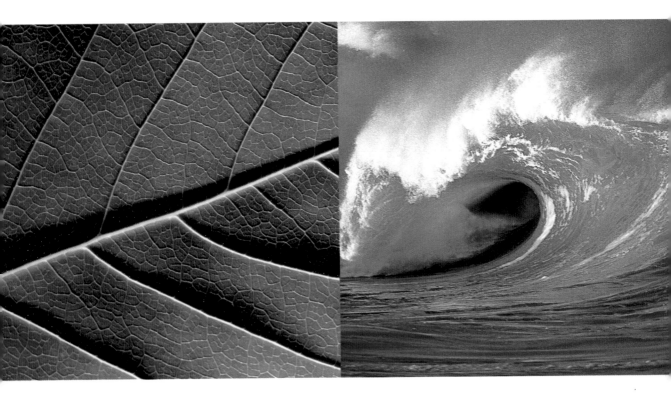

Fourth chakra –
The heart (centre of chest)

Colour of chakra: green or rose – encourages a strong love for others, can heal chest area, rose pink helps to encourage a soft, warm love

Can help: problems with expressing love, lack of sensitivity or connection with loved ones

During a full-body treatment, place a piece of paper or material in a green or rose pink colour over the solar plexus on the upper chest (see position 5, pages 44–45). Perform the reiki through the paper or material for 5 minutes, or until you feel enough energy has been taken in. Or you can visualize the colour going to the chakra as you channel the reiki.

Fifth chakra –
The throat (middle of throat)

Colour of chakra: turquoise blue – encourages you to speak the truth, strengthens your sensitive side, helps with issues of trust

Can help: inability to say what you feel, difficulty in communicating with others, not taking responsibility for life, throat problems

As part of a full-body treatment, place a turquoise-coloured piece of paper or material over the centre of the throat (see position 4, pages 42–43). Send the reiki through the paper or material for 5 minutes, or as long as you feel is needed. If you prefer, you can visualize the colour going to the chakra instead.

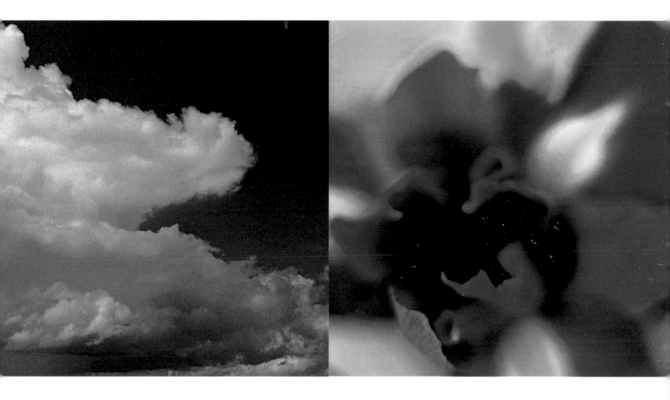

Sixth chakra –
The third eye (middle of forehead)
Colour of chakra: indigo – a spiritual colour, increases sense of respect and leadership qualities
Can help: tiredness, irritability, confused thoughts, mental stress, hay fever and insomnia

When performing a full-body treatment, place a piece of paper or material in an indigo colour over the middle of the forehead (see position 2, pages 38–39). Perform the reiki through the paper or material for 5 minutes, or until you feel the energy fading. Alternatively, as mentioned before you can visualize the colour flowing to the chakra as you channel the reiki energy.

Seventh chakra –
The crown (top of head)
Colour of chakra: purple, white and gold – promotes spiritual integration. White connects you to spiritual awareness, gold to your higher self
Can help: a lack of spirituality, a lack of trust in the higher self, angry rebellion about the way life is going

As part of a full-body treatment, place a piece of paper or material in purple, or white and gold as close to the top of the head as possible (see position 1, pages 36–37). Perform the reiki through the paper or material for 5 minutes, or for as long as is needed. You can also visualize the colour going to the chakra as you perform the reiki.

reiki and crystal healing

Crystals, like colour, have vibrational qualities which can be used for healing. Their powerful energies can be harnessed to focus on a specific blockage in a chakra or the aura, helping to remove it and, hopefully, preventing the onset of illness. They cannot, however, take away the negative emotions that can bring about illness in the first place; only reiki can work on these. When crystals are combined with reiki, the healing can be substantially increased, helping the imbalanced area to recover more quickly.

All crystals have their own individual qualities and have to be chosen carefully to work with the relevant chakra. The vibrational colour of the crystal usually relates to the colour that is associated with the chakra. For example, the wonderful healing stone, pink rose quartz, is used on the heart chakra, the colours of which are rose pink and green. Some people are comfortable with placing the crystal on the chakra and then transmitting the reiki energy through it. However, it is not known how the reiki energy is affected or possibly distorted by the energy of the crystal, so it is safer to place the stone on the chakra area and to perform the reiki on either side of the crystal, but *not* through it.

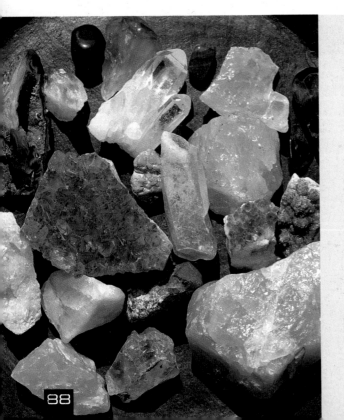

Cleansing crystals

When you use crystals as part of a reiki treatment, they will absorb negative energy from people so you should cleanse them before and after every treatment. Hold the crystals under running tap water for about 5 minutes, then dry them gently with a cloth. If the session was an especially emotional one, soak the crystal afterwards for 24 hours. They can also be laid in the sun for a day to energize them. Beware of soaking lapis lazuli as it is porous and will crumble; only rinse malachite in cool water; do not soak turquoise – re-energize it by performing reiki over it to cleanse it and do not put amethyst or rose quartz in the sun as they may fade.

crystals and their properties

CHAKRA	COLOUR	IMBALANCE	CRYSTAL BENEFIT	CRYSTALS TO USE
First chakra – the root	Red	Lack of fun, vitality or spontaneity	Strength, power, stabilizes and encourages optimism, purifying	Geode agate, tiger's eye, bloodstone
Second chakra – the sacral	Orange	Insecurity, self-doubts, confusion	Self-confidence, courage, grounding energy	Calcite, carnelian, tiger's eye
Third chakra – the solar plexus	Yellow	Fear, stress, tension, negativity	Happiness, stimulation, clear thinking, calming	Citrine, rose quartz, malachite
Fourth chakra – the heart	Green or rose	Selfishness, jealousy, lack of tenderness or compassion	Healing, balance, unconditional love, emotional wellbeing, loyalty	Rose quartz, aventurine, emerald
Fifth chakra – the throat	Turquoise blue	Nervousness, restlessness, problems with expressing feelings	Peace, serenity helps self-expression, aids communication and relieves stress	Lapis lazuli, turquoise, aquamarine
Sixth chakra – the third eye	Indigo	Lack of decisiveness, blockages, poor intuition	Intuition, awareness, transforming, objectivity	Amethyst, fluorite, sodalite
Seventh chakra – the crown	Purple, white and gold	Boredom, lack of spiritual growth, feelings of despair	Creativity, enlightenment, spiritual awareness (purple) purity, protection, helps meditation (white), wisdom (gold)	Clear quartz, amethyst, milky quartz

treating the chakras with reiki and crystal energy

First chakra – The root (base of spine)
HEALING STONES

Geode agate: This stone can enhance our sense of purpose, bring joy back into our lives and boost self-esteem.

Tiger's eye: A crystal that boosts creativity and concentrates energy.

Bloodstone: A purifying stone, it helps to increase optimism and boost inherent talents and decision making.

If someone is suffering from a lack of vitality or joy in their life (see chart), place one of these crystals on their lower pelvic region during a full-body treatment (see position 8, pages 50–51). Place your hands on their body, either side of the stone, and treat for 5 minutes as usual, letting the healing energies of the stone aid the person's recovery. To treat yourself, hold one of the stones in one hand, place the other one on your pelvic region and focus on the stone for 5 minutes.

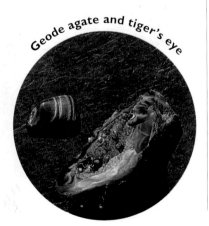
Geode agate and tiger's eye

Second chakra – The sacral (pelvic area)
HEALING STONES

Calcite: This stone can help build confidence, regain a lost identity and aid psychic development.

Carnelian: A crystal that helps to remove apathy, providing energy and motivation.

Tiger's eye: In the sacral chakra, this stone encourages wellbeing, optimism and basic inner strength.

To balance someone suffering from insecurity and a lack of confidence (see chart), place one of the above crystals on their pelvic area during a full-body treatment (see position 7, pages 48–49). Place your hands on their body on either side of the stone and treat for 5 minutes, letting the crystal work with the reiki. To treat yourself, choose a stone and hold in one hand. Place the other one on your pelvic area, close your eyes and concentrate on the stone for 5 minutes.

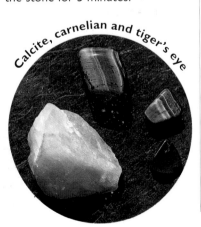
Calcite, carnelian and tiger's eye

Third chakra – The solar plexus (upper abdomen)
HEALING STONES

Citrine: Removes fear, calms and cleanses, creates a sense of worth.

Rose quartz: A very healing and comforting stone that encourages happiness and helps reduce the stress often stored in this area.

Malachite: A soothing crystal, it also brings inner peace and is also a good anti-depressant.

To reduce fear, tension or stress (see chart), place one of these crystals on their upper abdomen during a full-body treatment (see position 6, pages 46–47). Place your hands on their body on either side of the stone and treat for 5 minutes, letting the crystal dispel any restricting tension. To treat yourself, hold your stone in one hand, while putting the other one on your upper abdomen. Relax for 5 minutes, focusing on the stone.

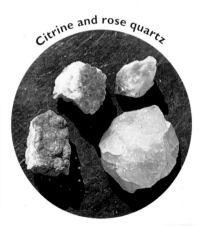
Citrine and rose quartz

Fourth chakra – The heart (centre of chest)
HEALING STONES

Rose quartz: Symbolizes love and, in the heart chakra, it helps us to support others emotionally and to give and receive unconditional love.
Aventurine: A calming stone that helps with mental and emotional imbalances, promoting wellbeing.
Emerald: A crystal that promotes loyalty and compassion for other people, reducing self interest. It also encourages romantic love.

To help remove jealousy and selfishness and to inspire love and compassion (see chart), place a crystal on the middle of their chest over the heart during a full-body treatment (see position 5, pages 44–45). Place your hands on their chest on either side of the stone and treat for 5 minutes, allowing the crystal to encourage feelings of love. To treat yourself, hold your chosen stone in one hand, and place the other one on the centre of your chest. Hold for 5 minutes, letting loving feelings emerge.

Fifth chakra – The throat (middle of throat)
HEALING STONES

Lapis lazuli: This stone aids mental and spiritual cleansing and encourages self expression.
Turquoise: A crystal that balances the mind, regulates the nervous system and aids communication.
Aquamarine: Helps to reduce fears and phobias and encourages good communication.

To dispel nervous and restless feelings and to encourage self-expression (see chart), place one of the crystals listed above on the centre of their throat during a full-body treatment (see position 4, pages 42–43). Place your hands on their throat on either side of the stone and treat for 5 minutes, allowing the crystal to clear communication blockages. To treat yourself, hold your throat crystal in one hand, and place other one on your throat. Hold for 5 minutes, allowing the throat chakra to draw energy and strengthen.

Sixth chakra – The third eye (middle of forehead)
HEALING STONES

Amethyst: This stone helps to absorb any negative emotions, it can be transformational, changing states of consciousness.
Fluorite: A crystal that can remove emotional blockages and help you to move on mentally.
Sodalite: Helps you to realize the purpose of your life, it is a stone that gives objectivity and new perspectives.

To remove blockages and help with lack of decisiveness (see chart), place a crystal on the middle of their forehead during a full-body treatment (see position 2, pages 38–39). Sit behind the person and place your hands on their forehead (temples) on either side of the stone and treat for 5 minutes, letting the crystal clear negative blockages. To treat yourself, hold your third eye stone in one hand, and place the other one on the third eye. Hold for 5 minutes.

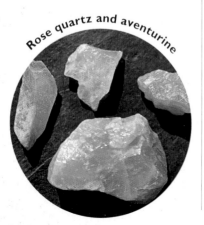

Rose quartz and aventurine

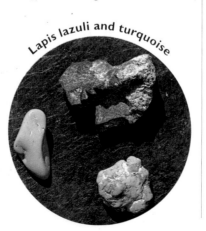

Lapis lazuli and turquoise

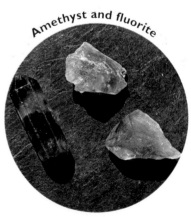

Amethyst and fluorite

Seventh chakra – The crown (top of head)
HEALING STONES

Clear quartz: A powerful, versatile crystal that helps to create balance, aids meditation and makes you realize the possibilities in life.

Amethyst: In this chakra, this promotes spiritual awareness and calms the mind, removing negative feelings and creating contentment.

Milky quartz: A stone that removes resentments and despair, it is very grounding.

To encourage spiritual growth and remove feelings of despair (see chart), place the crystal on the top of their head during a full-body treatment (see position 1, pages 36–37). Sitting behind the person, place your hands on their temples on either side of the stone and treat for 5 minutes, letting the crystal balance them and bring spiritual harmony and awareness. To treat yourself, hold your crown stone in one hand, and place the other hand on the crown of your head and hold for 5 minutes.

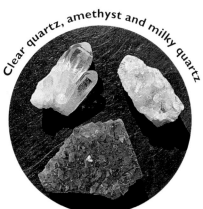

Clear quartz, amethyst and milky quartz

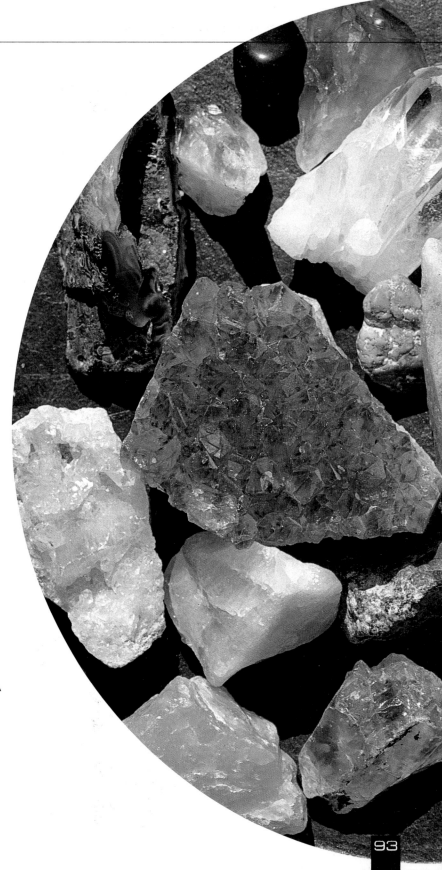

Further reading

Abundance through Reiki
Paula Horan, Lotus Light Publications,
USA 1995

Healing Reiki
Eleanor McKenzie, Hamlyn 1998

Living Reiki – Takata's teachings
as told by, Fran Brown, Life Rhythm,
USA 1992

Practical Reiki
Mari Hall, Thorsons 1997

Principles of Reiki
Kajsa Krishni Boräng, Thorsons 1997

Reiki
Chris and Penny Parkes, Vermilion 1998

Reiki
Penelope Quest, Piatkus 1999

Reiki for First Aid
Walter Lubeck, Lotus Light Publications,
USA 1995

Useful addresses

The Reiki Association
2 Manor Cottages
Stockley Hill, Peterchurch
Hereford, HR2 0SS, UK
Tel: 01981 550829 (10am–2pm)
Email: reikiassoc_office@compuserve.com

The Reiki School
Budworth, Shay Lane
Hale, Altrincham, WA15 8UE, UK
Tel: 0161 980 6453
Email:reikischool@mydtic.dircon.co.uk
www.selfpower.com/reikischool

The Reiki Alliance
PO Box 41, Cataldo
Idaho 83810–1041, USA
Tel: 208 783 3535
Fax: 208 783 4848

The Reiki Alliance
Honthorstraat 41 11
1071 DG Amsterdam
Netherlands
Tel: 31 20 67 19 276
Fax: 31 20 67 11 736

Office of the Grand Master
Pl Box 220, Cataldo
Idaho 83810, USA
Tel: 208 682 9009
Fax: 208 682 9567

Reiki Outreach International
c/o Soyin Tang,
17 Brincliffe Crescent,
Sheffield, S11 9AW, UK
Tel: 0114 255 2927

Reiki Outreach International
Mary MacFayden
Po Box 609, Fair Oaks
California 95628, USA
Tel: 916 863 1500
Fax: 916 863 6464

**The International Center for Reiki
Training**
21421 Hilltop #28
Southfield, Michigan 48034 USA
Tel: 800 332 8112/248 948 8112
Email: reikicent@aol.com
www.reiki.org

Author's Acknowledgements

My grateful thanks to Liz Dean at Collins & Brown for encouraging me to write this book, to my editor Muna Reyal for her helpful assistance, to Sue Miller for her great design and Winfried Heinze for his wonderful photography. Also thanks to Chris Parkes, my reiki master and consultant, for all his guidance and to all my friends, particularly Steve, for supporting and encouraging me while I wrote this book.

The author and publishers would like to thank the following organizations for the loan of props and accessories:

Take Ltd
182 Upper Richmond Road West
London SW14 8AW
020 8876 9216

Virgo Bodywork Tables
Rowleys Yard, Woodlands Park Road,
London N15 3RT
020 8802 5008

Neal Street East
5 Neal Street, Covent Garden
London WC2H 9PU
020 7240 0135

Muji
Head Office
4th Floor, 167–169 Great Portland Street
London WIN 5FD
020 7323 2208

Prices Candles
110 York Road
London SW11 3RU
020 7801 2030